Juicing
for Health

Juicing
for Health

CAROLINE WHEATER

Thorsons

Thorsons
An Imprint of HarperCollins*Publishers*
77–85 Fulham Palace Road,
Hammersmith, London W6 8JB

The Thorsons website address is www.thorsons.com

First published by Thorsons 1993
This edition published by Thorsons 2001

10 9 8 7 6 5 4

Text illustrations by Helen Holroyd

A catalogue record for this book
is available from the British Library

ISBN 0 00 710691 2

Printed and bound in Great Britain by
Martins the Printers Ltd, Berwick upon Tweed

To Simon

acknowledgements

Thanks first of all to Leon Chaitow, Kathryn Marsden and Simon Brown for valuable nutritional advice. Special thanks must go to the following people: Sarah Zebaida of Squeeze Us, Pineapple West Studios, central London, and Paul Martin, owner and barman extraordinaire of Kudos Cocktail Bar, in Kew, west London, for providing wonderful juicy recipes for inclusion in Chapter 8, the Fresh Juice Bar; also to Anne Sheasby, consultant home economist, for devising the juice pulp recipes in Chapter 9, Pulper's Paradise. Sarah, Paul and Anne, I couldn't have done it without your help! Gratitude to both Kenwood and Braun UK Ltd for providing juicers for testing purposes. And finally a big thank you to Sarah Sutton, my Editor at Thorsons, for all her encouragement during 1992.

contents

Introduction   xi

Part 1: The Wonders of Juice   1
Raw Juice Secrets   2
The Juice Kitchen   9
Prepare to Juice   15

Part 2: Beauty, Peak Health and Vitality   48
Juices for Beauty   51
Juices for Health   60
Living with Added Zest   89
Detox and Revitalize   103

Part 3: Juice it Up!   124
The Fresh Juice Bar   125
Pulper's Paradise   166

Appendix 1: Glossary – Vitamins and Minerals   191
Appendix 2: Useful Information   201
Further Reading   206
Index   208

introduction
the fresh facts

Every time I sip a fresh fruit or vegetable juice, I'm amazed by the flavour, the colour, the texture. To me, fresh juices are everything a healthy food should be: all-natural, bursting with taste, and choc-full of good things, from vitamins and minerals to enzymes and inner cleansers. It was back in 1992 that I first came across the health phenomenon that has since swept Europe, the States and Australia. A young woman named Sarah Zebaida had been so impressed with the fresh juices she'd come across while travelling in Asia that she'd opened Britain's first ever juice bar – Squeeze Us at the Pineapple Dance Studios in central London.

It was a revelation. Just a few sips of her myriad blends and I was hooked – the fruitiest fruit juices; the zestiest vegetable juices; rich smoothies that were just as filling as a light lunch. Since then, of course, there's been no looking back and juice bars everywhere are doing a roaring trade.

Of course, you don't have to go out to benefit from this healthiest of trends; juices are easy to make at home. All you need is a juicer and a shopping list – full of your favourite fruits and vegetables. Juicing is surprisingly quick and immensely satisfying to do and can be done all year round as you make use of seasonal varieties. Root vegetable juices can be just as tasty as fruity ones – and if you don't believe me, pop a parsnip in to juice ... or a carrot ... or a tomato. Smoothies are the ultimate in comfort juices, drink one just before going to bed for a solid night's sleep.

In short, freshly juiced juices are sweeter, more piquant, more tart, more creamy, more flavoursome, more varied than anything you might ever have tasted before. And because the fruits and vegetables you choose to use go straight from your shopping basket into your juicer and into you, you'll get maximum benefit from their rainbow coalition of vitamins and minerals. Bearing in mind that the latest healthy eating advice is to consume at least five portions of fruit and vegetables a day, juicing makes perfect sense. It won't of course provide you with all-important fibre (that's why you need to eat whole fruit and vegetables too) but it will ensure you're getting a wide range of vital nutrients. Investing a little extra time and money brings huge dividends to your wellbeing.

Which is why juicing is a habit that deserves to be got. In my comprehensive guide, you'll find out why fresh juices really are so special and how to go about making them. Not to mention hundreds of recipes for health, beauty and vitality, a detox plan, recipes for left-over pulp, and easy-to-understand nutritional notes about each fruit and vegetable included.

As I discovered all those years ago, tasting is believing – so why not try juicing for yourself.

the wonders of juice

raw juice secrets

With the fast pace of modern life, it's easy to get caught up in the clutches of convenience, and to forget the simple and natural things in life. While we're all aware of the benefits, eating fresh food is something that's often pushed to the bottom of our priority list. We make time to see friends, play sport and clean the house, but when it comes to supplying energy and nutrition through the best sorts of food it's usually another story.

Lately we have become used to supplementing our diets with vitamin and mineral pills, as a kind of insurance policy. Supplements have their place and can be very effective, but they can't take the place of a diet full of natural, health-giving foods. Fresh fruit and vegetable juices are part of the all-natural line-up that can knock spots off convenience products. Not only do they provide a wealth of vitamins, minerals and other nutrients, they are also cleansing and balancing for the body as a whole; the equivalent of a multivitamin pill in a glass, with hidden benefits.

RAW HEALTH

Once you have tasted your own fresh fruit and vegetable juices you'll realize that there is little comparison between the liquid that flows from your juicer and that which flows from shop-bought cartons. Most readymade juices rely on concentrated juice and extra water to bulk them up. Look on the label and you'll find that some juices contain additives such as sugar, colours, flavours and preservatives too, while the latest range of freshly juiced juices are wildly expensive.

Homemade juices have nothing added, nothing taken away, just 100 per cent pure juice. The fruits and vegetables which you choose to juice will be as fresh as possible and will not have undergone any processing. This makes a real difference, as any sort of cooking reduces the content of vitamins and minerals, and sometimes destroys them altogether.

Every time you drink a glass of juice it will contain virtually the same amount of nutrients (although not as much fibre) as if you were eating the fruit or vegetable whole. In fact, you will probably be absorbing far more, as it takes quite a bit of produce to make just one 8 fl oz/230ml glass of juice. For example, you would have to eat 2 apples, or 3 carrots, or nearly a whole pineapple to consume the quantity of nutrients that goes into 8fl oz/230ml of juice.

THE PIONEERS

Of course, like most 'novel' ideas, the concept of juicing is not new at all. Since the nineteenth century, doctors and naturopaths have been treating patients with fresh juices and raw foods to help improve their health. Germany and Switzerland are together regarded as the cradle of the therapy, and during the nineteenth and early part of the twentieth centuries nurtured a number of famous pioneers, such as Father Kniepp, Dr Kellog, Dr Max Bircher-Benner and Dr Max Gerson. Between them they developed the *Röhsaft Kur* (the fresh juice cure), which is still practised today at health clinics all over the world. American pioneers, such as the late Dr Norman Walker, and Ann Wigmore, founder of the Hippocrates Health Institute in Boston, have continued their work. There is simply masses of research and practice to draw upon. For many years, therefore, juices have been used by naturopaths in Europe and America to help treat a whole range of minor, and sometimes major, ailments. It's no surprise when you consider what a rich source of nutrients and cleansing elements they are.

VITAMINS AND MINERALS

Fresh juices are packed with many of the vitamins and minerals that keep us well. As with all natural, whole foods, the vitamins and minerals in fruit and vegetables are often bound on to other nutrients that help absorption. For example, bioflavonoids are found in the pith of citrus fruit, and they aid the absorption of vitamin C. The minerals found in fresh produce are chelated to amino acids, or sometimes a vitamin, to make them easier to absorb.

The list below reveals the range of vitamins and minerals in fresh juices; beta carotene, vitamin C, potassium and phosphorus are found at particularly high levels.

Vitamins

beta-carotene (the vegetarian form of vitamin A)

vitamin B1 (thiamine)

vitamin B2 (riboflavin)

vitamin B3 (niacin)

vitamin B5 (pantothenic acid)

vitamin B6 (pyridoxine)

folic acid

biotin

choline

inositol

vitamin C

vitamin E

Minerals

calcium

chlorine

chromium

cobalt

copper

fluorine

iodine

iron

magnesium

manganese

phosphorus

potassium

selenium

sodium

sulphur

zinc

For more information on the nutrients contained in fresh juices, see chapters 4–6, and Appendix 1.

THE ANTIOXIDANTS

You may have heard of antioxidant nutrients in newspaper and magazine reports, and if you haven't you will soon. They are the focus of scores of research studies, which are looking at whether a group of vitamins and minerals – particularly vitamins A, C, E and selenium – can give protection against degenerative diseases such as cancer, heart disease, premature ageing and cataracts. Scientists believe that they may be the key to limiting the impact of these often devastating diseases.

Of course, fruits and vegetables are full of antioxidants – vitamins C and E – and juices made with them are naturally a very good source. The reason why these nutrients may have a revolutionary impact on our preventive healthcare is that they are able to quench unbalanced molecules, known as free radicals.

FREE RADICALS

Free radicals are generated by toxins, such as those produced by air pollution or smoke. They react with other molecules in our bodies and destabilize them, therefore putting cells at risk. They have been implicated in the development of diseases like cancer and heart disease, because they are capable of destroying other, healthy molecules, which in turn become unstable.

So, drinking plenty of fresh juices may have a long-term impact on your health, as well as perking you up in the short-term. For an antioxidant booster juice recipe, turn to Chapter 5.

EXTRA NUTRIENTS

Fresh juices also contain other substances which are not classified as vitamins or minerals, but which may be beneficial to our health. For example, plant pigments like carotenoids and anthocyanins; substances that combat plant viruses and bacteria; and compounds that create smell and taste. Current research is trying to establish just what these individual essences can do, but the suggestion is that they are an integral part of the goodness supplied by raw fruit and vegetables and their juices.

EASY TO DIGEST

Fruit and vegetable juices are easy to digest, and are ideal for people who can't cope with a lot of fibre, or who don't want to munch their way through a pound of carrots (remember fresh juices should not replace your dietary intake of whole fruits and vegetables, of which the fibre is essential for good digestion). Because they are liquids, fruit and vegetable juices are quickly digested in the stomach, and the nutrients absorbed into the bloodstream.

The digestive process is also helped by the presence of active plant enzymes, which join with the stomach's own enzymes in breaking down the juice. The efficiency of these workers enables nutrients to be absorbed into the body within minutes of being eaten. Plant enzymes also help to neutralize excess proteins and fat from other foods. Some, like papain from papaya and bromelain from pineapple, are especially good at calming indigestion.

SUPER CLEANSERS

Fresh juices have remarkable cleansing and restorative powers. To start with, fruits and vegetables all hold stores of pure water, which has been filtered and distilled through their complex structures. This means that the digestive system has one less set of impurities to deal with.

In addition, all fruits contain acid, which can help remove toxins from the digestive tract. Citrus fruits contain the strongest acid compound – citric acid – and other fruits contain the milder tartaric and malic acids. Some fruits, such as oranges and apples, also contain pectin, which can absorb fats and toxins from the digestive tract (as well as making jam and marmalade set).

Green vegetables are rich in chlorophyll (the substance that enables plants to harvest energy from the sunlight), which also has cleansing properties. That's why greens like watercress and spinach can be so helpful on a detox programme. Certain other vegetables, such as carrot and tomato, have a reputation for acting as tonics to the liver too. For further information on doing a detox programme with fresh juices, turn to Chapter 7.

KEEP THE BALANCE

Both fruit and vegetable juices are strong alkalizers once they have been digested, which is a plus point for most of us, because the average diet of too much protein and too many refined, processed foods creates over-acidity. Like any other living thing, the body has a subtle pH balance between acid and alkaline, tipping the scales in favour of alkaline. Drinking a glass of juice a day can help restore this essential balance.

A GOOD HEALTH GUARANTEE?

Juices on their own won't bring you perfect health, but they can contribute to it. To increase your chances of a long and healthy life, you might like to consider other beneficial changes you can make to your daily routine, such as:

- stop smoking
- cut back on alcohol
- take regular exercise
- cut down on animal fats (meat and dairy produce)
- increase consumption of fruit and vegetables
- drink 3–4 pints of water a day
- put time aside to relax – properly

SOME GOLDEN RULES

Beginners should limit their intake to up to three 8fl oz/230ml glasses of juice a day. Veterans can up the amount to six glasses.
Always dilute dark green vegetable juices (ie broccoli, spinach, watercress) and dark red vegetable juices (ie beetroot, red cabbage) by four parts to one. They are very potent in taste and effect.

Drink vegetable *and* fruit juices in order to get the maximum nutritional benefit. Too many fruit juices will overload your system with the fruit sugar, fructose.

Fruit juice causes a rapid rise in blood sugar, and anyone suffering from candidiasis should be cautious regarding excessive sugar intake. If you are prone to suffer from thrush, therefore, or suspect you may have a yeast infection in the digestive tract, you should take professional advice before increasing your intake of fruit juices (vegetable juices are, on the whole, not a problem in such cases). This advice also applies to anyone with low blood sugar or diabetes.

Avoid mixing vegetable and fruit juices together in the same glass or you may well suffer from a dose of flatulence! The exceptions are apple and carrot, which you can mix freely with any other juice.

See Chapter 8 for advice on children and juices.

the juice kitchen

Juicing is really a very simple improvement to add to your daily routine, and juicing at home is fun, easy, and economical. You can produce an almost endless variety of colourful fresh juices which are brimming with health-giving nutrients. But of course, before you can enjoy the bounty of fresh juices, you need to know how to make them. Here are the guidelines to help you equip your kitchen and get the most out of juicing.

HOW TO JUICE

The most essential piece of equipment for any juice novice is a juicing machine – this is not the same as a blender, liquidizer or food processor (although some food processors may have a juicing attachment). A juicer separates the juice from the fibrous pulp, creating a smooth liquid, whereas a blender or liquidizer simply purées both fibre and juice together. You can juice by hand (see page 11), but it's laborious to say the least!

Choosing a Juicer

To get the best value from your juicer, it should be able to juice most fruits and vegetables. You might be told that a juicer can't handle citrus fruits – but that's just because they won't turn out like the 'freshly squeezed' varieties you can buy in supermarkets. Instead they look much thicker and creamier, because they include the valuable white pith that surrounds the fruit. With a cheaper juicer you might have trouble juicing stringy produce like bean sprouts, alfalfa, parsley and wheatgrass – so if you want to be able to juice absolutely anything perfectly it's better to pay the premium for a more sophisticated model.

Make sure that whichever juicer you buy, it's easy to clean and simple to put together. There's nothing worse than facing a physical and mental assault course every time you fancy a juice.

Prices range from reasonable to very expensive, but if you're just starting out, it's probably wise to buy at the cheaper end of the range, just in case (and it's highly unlikely!) you discover juicing isn't for you. Investment in a better model is always possible later on. Let's see what's available.

Centrifugal Juicers

These models are at the lower end of the price scale and are made by companies such as Braun, Philips, Kenwood and Moulinex. They are electrically powered and work by grating fruits and vegetables, then spinning them rapidly to separate juice from fibrous pulp. The juice then runs through an outlet into a jug, and the pulp is ejected into a separate container. Centrifugal juicers cannot handle a huge amount of produce all at once, and must be kept clean, or they clog up with pulp. They produce thick, creamy juice and wet pulp (see Chapter 9 for pulp recipes). They are not as juice-efficient as some of the more sophisticated and expensive models.

Nose-Cone Pressure or Masticating Juicers

These models extract a greater quantity of juice from produce than centrifugal juicers because they put much more pressure on the fruits and vegetables. Rather than grating produce, they chop or churn it, then ram the resulting pulp into a mesh nose-cone from where the juice is forced out. Nose-cone juicers can be electrically or manually powered (when a lever system is incorporated). They tend to be able to cope better with the tougher produce such as rinds, stalks, and very hard vegetables; as a result they are usually more expensive than centrifugal models.

Hydraulic Juice Presses

Juice presses are the most efficient of all at extracting juice. This is because they can bring to bear the pressure of between three and five tons on your chosen fruits and vegetables. The press is brought down on the produce and the juice filters out through a fine cloth; the end pulp is reduced to a cardboard consistency (not much good for anything but compost). Hydraulic presses can be electrically powered or manual, but the former is extremely expensive. Nevertheless, the juice extracted from the press method is the most nutritionally complete of all the juices. They are available from specialist suppliers. See Appendix 2, specialist equipment.

Citrus Squeezers

If you really don't like the thick juice that a juicing machine produces from oranges, lemons, limes and grapefruit, then you can use a citrus squeezer for cleaner, thinner juice. You can buy a simple glass or plastic squeezer, or invest in an electric squeezer if you have trouble gripping the fruit tightly enough (those with arthritis or rheumatism may find electric models helpful).

Juicing by Hand

For hand juicing you'll need a grater, a bowl, a fine sieve and some muslin or specially designed juice cloths (see Appendix 2, specialist equipment). Here's how you do it:

1. Grate your chosen fruit or vegetable into a bowl.
2. Place the grated produce in the middle of a square piece of muslin (or juice cloth). Gather the edges into a bundle, and squeeze the contents hard over a bowl.
3. For an extra filtration process, tip the juice through a fine sieve into a bowl. It is then ready to drink.

Other Equipment

Once you have your juicer, you will probably need and find useful:

- a hard-bristle scrubbing brush to remove dirt from vegetable and fruit skins about to be juiced
- weighing scales to measure out produce
- a chopping board
- a sharp knife, capable of cutting very hard vegetables
- a peeler
- a plastic/glass measuring jug indicating millilitres and fluid ounces
- a large jug for storing juice
- cling film to keep stored juice airtight
- a blender for mixing juices with fruit purées, yoghurt, milk, water, honey and other extras (see Chapter 8).
- a fine mesh sieve for straining juice if it seems 'bitty'
- an apron to avoid splashing your clothes with vividly coloured juice

Cleaning While Juicing

if you are making a lot of juice, clean the juicer once or twice under running water to remove unnecessary pulp. If you have put a very pungent or colourful fruit or vegetable through the juicer, run a little water through the opening to cleanse the innards of the machine, or chop up some apple and put that through the juicer. Both these methods prevent subsequent juices from being discoloured or tasting odd.

Looking After Your Juicer

Once you have finished with your juicer for the day, make sure it is scrupulously clean and dry, or you may get bugs making the pulp container into a comfy home. Every once in a while give it a thorough clean with a little bleach, to rid the plastic of any juice stains that might have collected. Alternatively, use a solution of bicarbonate of soda diluted in a small bowl of water. The better you treat your juicer, the longer it will last.

JUICE TIPS

Here are some tips to help you make the most of your juicing. They are simple but essential points of which you should be aware.

The Fresher the Better

Fresh juices should preferably be drunk just after they have been made, or during the same day. This ensures that they contain the maximum number of nutrients. Some vitamins are especially vulnerable to fresh air and can be destroyed in a matter of hours on exposure to it. If you are going to keep your juice, store it in the refrigerator in an airtight container or a Thermos flask.

Taste the Difference

The consistency and flavour of fresh juices is very different from juices you can buy in the shops. They may seem odd at first, but you'll soon begin to prefer the texture and taste of juices made at home. They can be very thick, and are always much stronger-tasting than you will be used to. Some of them can look rather an odd colour (e.g. potato, grape, orange), and some of them are so vivid (e.g. red cabbage, red pepper, strawberries) you won't be able to take your eyes off them! The key is to stay open-minded and not turn up your nose at natural fruit juices just because they don't look or taste like the processed, packaged juices which are more familiar.

Unpalatability

If you find that certain juices really do taste unpalatable, try adding them to a *ready-warmed* soup or stew, to mask the flavour (cooking the juice will remove some of the nutrients).

Dilution

Children should always drink juices diluted, but if adults prefer them that way that's fine too. You can dilute juices with still or sparkling water, milk, soda, even lemonade — however, you'll find them easiest on the digestive system if you just use still water.

BUYING FRESH FRUITS AND VEGETABLES

What to Look For

Produce bought for juicing should be as fresh and as high a quality as your budget will stretch to, ensuring a better-tasting and more nutritionally complete juice. Watch out for mature and ripe produce, which will contain more vitamins and minerals. For example, although the mature outer leaves of a cabbage or lettuce may look unappealing, they contain the most nutrients and are therefore very valuable in juicing terms — just think, you won't actually have to chew on a leaf! The riper, more mature fruits and vegetables will also be easier to juice, and easier for your stomach to digest. Avoid buying produce that looks as though it has been sitting around for too long, is bruised, going droopy, or losing its colour. Juicing uses up a lot of fruit and vegetables, so it's probably best to do a bulk buy every three or four days to stock up on juicing ingredients.

The Benefits of Organic

Organic fruit and vegetables tend to be more expensive than standard varieties, but are now widely available. But why choose organic? First of all, their proponents say that they taste better, and second comes the reassuring fact that they have not been exposed to any chemical treatments. No chemical fertilizers, pesticides, herbicides or growth inhibitors (used while produce is in storage or transportation). This means that there will be no chemical residues, however small, lurking in the skin or outer layer of the produce. In addition, organic produce is not waxed; standard cucumbers, oranges and lemons often are. Organic produce often seems much riper too.

If a fruit or vegetable has thick rind or skin it doesn't really make much difference, because the residues won't penetrate the inner flesh, and you will probably have to remove the rind/skin to juice the contents. The problem comes with thin-skinned produce like carrots, cucumbers, peaches and apples, which we might scrub, but don't usually peel. We could be ingesting an invisible layer of chemicals and wax without even realizing it. So why not peel everything? The best reason is that a significant amount of nutrients usually lie in the thin peel, and we would lose out by throwing it away. Buying organic means that you don't have to worry about any of this and can juice whichever peel you like.

Now let's look at some practical tips on which fruit and vegetables to buy and how to prepare them for juicing.

prepare to juice

Juicing is a bit like a voyage of discovery, and it's the kind of activity that you can easily adapt to your own likes and dislikes. Here are descriptions of a range of fresh juices, including how to prepare the fruit and vegetables, their vitamin and mineral content, and an approximate calorie count per 100g of each fruit and vegetable (equivalent to 3–4fl oz/80–115ml of juice). You can enjoy these juices on their own, or try out the recipes beginning in Chapter 4, as you please.

FRUIT

Apple

Apple goes well with just about anything, or enjoy it as a single juice. It has a lovely flavour, a brownish colour if you use the pips, and is quite sweet. It is the only fruit juice that can happily be mixed with any vegetable juice.

PREPARATION
Cut into quarters; removing core is optional. Do not peel.

VITAMINS
Rich in beta-carotene, folic acid, C, small amounts of B1, B2, B3, B6, biotin and E.

MINERALS
Rich in calcium, chlorine, magnesium, phosphorus, potassium, sulphur, small amounts of copper and zinc.

Apricot

Light orange in colour, apricot has a summery aroma — and is a delicious sweet mixer.
Tastes and looks lovely with frothy lemonade.

PREPARATION
Cut in half and take out stone. Do not peel.

VITAMINS
Rich in beta-carotene, B3, B5, folic acid, C, small amounts of B1, B2, B6.

MINERALS
Rich in calcium, magnesium, phosphorus, potassium, sulphur, small amounts of copper,
iron and zinc.

CALORIES PER 100G
28

Avocado

Avocado does not juice well, because its flesh is too oily. However, it does make an
excellent blender, to be mixed with other fruit juices, especially if you want a high-energy
drink.

PREPARATION
Simply chop in half, peel away outer skin and remove stone. Then mash and blend with
juice.

VITAMINS
Rich in beta-carotene, B3, B5, folic acid, biotin, C, E, small amounts of B1, B2, B6.

Rich in calcium, magnesium, phosphorus, potassium, sulphur, small amounts of copper and iron.

CALORIES PER 100G
223

Banana

Banana juice is absolutely delicious, with a creamy consistency. Unfortunately, it's terribly wasteful – you only get a dribble of juice from a whole banana. As with avocado, it's better to blend it mashed with other more easily obtained juices.

PREPARATION
Peel and mash, ready to blend with juice.

VITAMINS
Rich in in beta-carotene, B3, folic acid, C, small amounts of B1, B2, B6, E.

MINERALS
Rich in calcium, chlorine, magnesium, phosphorus, potassium, sulphur, small amounts of copper, iron, manganese and zinc.

CALORIES PER 100G
79

Blackberry

Sweet, dark purple and pungent, a lovely mixer juice for an autumnal cocktail. Free, too, if you can pick fresh blackberries from the hedgerow.

PREPARATION
None needed – just a quick rinse under the tap.

Rich in beta-carotene, C, E, small amounts of biotin, B1, B2, B3, B5, B6.

MINERALS
Rich in calcium, chlorine, magnesium, phosphorus, potassium, sulphur, sodium, small amounts of copper and iron.

CALORIES PER 100G
29

Blackcurrant

One of the sweetest berries around, with a raw-cane sugar taste. A good mixer but too strong to be drunk on its own.

PREPARATION
Remove stalks, rinse currants. Do not chop or peel.

VITAMINS
Rich in beta-carotene, biotin, C, E, small amounts of B1, B2, B3, B5, B6.

MINERALS
Rich in calcium, chlorine, magnesium, phosphorus, potassium, sodium, sulphur, small amounts of copper and iron.

CALORIES PER 100G
28

Blueberry

Refreshingly sweet and dark purple in colour, a delicious juice that blends well with other berries and tastes great in Smoothies.

PREPARATION
None needed – just a quick rinse under the tap.

Rich in vitamin B1, B2, B6, C, biotin and folic acid.

MINERALS

Calcium, chromium, magnesium.

CALORIES PER 100G

86

Cherry

Depending on the ripeness and type of the cherry, colour ranges from dark red to purple — a delicious addition to any fruit juice combination.

PREPARATION

A bit time-consuming but worth it in the end. Chop in half and de-stone. Do not peel. Alternatively invest in a mechanical cherry-stoner.

VITAMINS

Rich in beta-carotene, folic acid, C, small amounts of biotin, B1, B2, B3, B5, B6, E.

MINERALS

Rich in calcium, magnesium, phosphorus, potassium, sodium, sulphur, small amounts of copper, iron, manganese and zinc.

CALORIES PER 100G

47

Cranberry

This scarlet juice tastes very tart on its own, but it is a great mixer, especially in cocktails. It's a useful treatment for cystitis.

PREPARATION

Simply rinse.

Rich in beta-carotene, folic acid, C, small amounts of B1, B2, B3, B5, B6.

MINERALS
Rich in calcium, chlorine, magnesium, phosphorus, potassium, sodium, sulphur, small amounts of copper and iron.

CALORIES PER 100G
15

Gooseberry

A slightly tart juice, light green in colour, great for mixing with sweeter varieties.

PREPARATION
None, simply rinse.

VITAMINS
Rich in beta-carotene, C, small amounts of B1, B2, B3, B5, B6, E.

MINERALS
Rich in calcium, chlorine, magnesium, phosphorus, potassium, sulphur, small amounts of copper, iron, manganese and zinc.

CALORIES PER 100G
37

Grape

Grape juice has a lovely sweet, tangy taste. It's quite thick, and has a pale green or dark pink colour.

PREPARATION
Pluck away from woody stalks, rinse. Do not remove pips.

VITAMINS
Rich in C, E, small amounts of B1, B2, B3.

MINERALS
Rich in calcium, magnesium, phosphorus, potassium, sodium, sulphur, small amounts of copper, iron and zinc.

CALORIES PER 100G
60

Grapefruit

A smooth, slightly tart juice, pale in colour and creamy in texture. Pink grapefruit juice is slightly sweeter and is tinged with a rosy colour. Great on its own or mixed.

PREPARATION
Remove peel, but not pith. Cut into chunks.

VITAMINS
Rich in beta-carotene, folic acid, C, small amounts of B1, B2, B3, B5, B6, E.

MINERALS
Rich in calcium, magnesium, phosphorus, potassium, small amounts of copper, iron, manganese and zinc.

CALORIES PER 100G
32

Greengage

A grass-green colour, sweet and plummy taste.

PREPARATION
Cut in half and remove stone.

Rich in folic acid, C, small amounts of B1, B2, B3, B5, B6, E.

MINERALS
Rich in calcium, chlorine, magnesium, phosphorus, potassium, sodium, sulphur, small amounts of copper, iron and zinc.

CALORIES PER 100G
47

Guava

A tropical-tasting juice, from a tropical fruit. Creamy, green juice, lovely in cocktails. Do not remove seeds.

PREPARATION
Peel and chop into chunks.

VITAMINS
Rich in beta-carotene B3, C, small amounts of B1, B2, B5, B6.

MINERALS
Rich in calcium, magnesium, phosphorus, potassium, sodium, small amounts of copper, iron, manganese and zinc.

CALORIES PER 100G
51

Kiwi Fruit

A wonderful lime-green colour, zesty-tasting juice – a good mixer.

PREPARATION
Peel away skin, cut flesh into quarters.

Rich in beta-carotene, C, small amounts of B1, B2, B3.

MINERALS

Rich in calcium, magnesium, phosphorus, potassium, sodium, small amount of iron.

CALORIES PER 100G

61

Lemon

A very sharp juice of a creamy, pale yellow colour. Only use in small amounts as a mixer.

PREPARATION

Peel away skin, chop into chunks. Remove pips if you prefer.

VITAMINS

Rich in C, small amounts of B1, B2, B3, B5, B6, and biotin.

MINERALS

Rich in calcium, chlorine, magnesium, phosphorus, potassium, sodium, sulphur, small amounts of copper and iron.

CALORIES PER 100G

15

Lime

Sharp juice like lemon, but slightly sweeter. Again you only need a small amount as a mixer.

PREPARATION

Peel away skin, chop into chunks. Remove pips if preferred.

Rich in beta-carotene, folic acid, C, small amounts of B1, B2, B3, B5.

MINERALS

Rich in calcium, phosphorus, potassium, sodium, small amounts of copper, iron and zinc.

CALORIES PER 100G

30

Mango

A very thick, orange juice, goes extremely well with pineapple and banana. Needs to be mixed because it is so thick. I prefer organic mangoes, they seem to be riper and more juicy.

PREPARATION

Cut in half, remove flat stone, scoop flesh from casing with a spoon.

VITAMINS

Rich in beta-carotene, C, small amounts of B1, B2, B3, B5, B6.

MINERALS

Rich in calcium, magnesium, phosphorus, potassium, sodium, small amounts of copper, iron, manganese and zinc.

CALORIES PER 100G

65

Melon (orange, yellow)

This juice is refreshing and aromatic, but should only be drunk on its own. This is because it goes through the digestive system quicker than any other fruit and would restrict the absorption of nutrients from other juices.

Cut into quarters, remove flesh from rind in chunks. You can juice the seeds or remove them. You can juice the rind if you want to – make sure it's clean.

VITAMINS
Rich in beta-carotene, folic acid, C, small amounts of B1, B2, B3, B5, B6, E.

MINERALS
Rich in calcium, chlorine, magnesium, phosphorus, potassium, sodium, sulphur, small amounts of copper, iron and zinc.

CALORIES PER 100G
21

Nectarine

A lovely peachy taste and colour, refreshing and wonderful combined with berry juices.

PREPARATION
Cut into quarters, remove stone. Do not peel.

VITAMINS
Rich in beta-carotene, folic acid, C, small amounts of B1, B2, B3, B5, B6.

MINERALS
Rich in calcium, magnesium, phosphorus, potassium, small amounts of copper, iron, manganese and zinc.

CALORIES PER 100G
49

Orange

A great-tasting, all-round juice; comes out yellow instead of orange because of the white pith. Good on its own or can be mixed.

Peel, cut into chunks.

VITAMINS
Rich in beta-carotene, C, small amounts of B1, B2, B3, B5, B6, E.

MINERALS
Rich in calcium, magnesium, phosphorus, potassium, small amounts of copper, iron, manganese and zinc.

CALORIES PER 100G
46

Papaya

Like mango, a very thick juice, which needs to be diluted with a lighter type like apple or pineapple. Deep pink colour.

PREPARATION
Cut in half, scoop out seeds (or leave them in if preferred), scoop out flesh with a spoon.

VITAMINS
Rich in beta-carotene, C, small amounts of B1, B2, B3, B5, B6.

MINERALS
Rich in calcium, magnesium, phosphorus, potassium, sodium, small amounts of copper, iron, manganese and zinc.

CALORIES PER 100G
39

Passion Fruit

A dark brown juice with a sweet taste.

Peel and scoop out flesh.

Rich in beta-carotene, B3, C, small amount of B2.

Rich in calcium, chlorine, magnesium, phosphorus, potassium, sodium, sulphur, small amount of iron.

34

Peach

Nectar of the Gods! Sweet, flowery aroma, orange juice.

Cut in half, remove stone. Do not peel.

Rich in beta-carotene, folic acid, B3, C, small amounts of biotin, B1, B2, B5, B6.

Rich in calcium, magnesium, phosphorus, potassium, sulphur, sodium, small amounts of copper, iron and zinc.

33

Pear

A versatile juice which goes with most others, milder tasting and less thick than some.

Remove stalk, cut in quarters lengthways. Do not peel or remove pips.

VITAMINS
Rich in beta-carotene, folic acid, C, small amounts of B1, B2, B3, B5, B6.

MINERALS
Rich in calcium, magnesium, phosphorus, potassium, small amounts of copper, iron, manganese and zinc.

CALORIES PER 100G
59

Pineapple

Lovely, sweet taste, very palatable amber juice, either on its own or mixed with others. Contains bromelain.

PREPARATION
Cut into rings, remove outer spiny skin. Cut into chunks.

VITAMINS
Rich in beta-carotene, folic acid, C, small amounts of B1, B2, B3, B5, B6.

MINERALS
Rich in calcium, magnesium, phosphorus, potassium, sodium, small amounts of copper, iron and zinc.

CALORIES PER 100G
49

Plum

Golden red colour, sweet and aromatic, goes well with any berry juice, or milder juice.

Cut in half, remove stone. Do not peel.

VITAMINS
Rich in beta-carotene, folic acid, C, small amounts of B1, B2, B5, B6, E.

MINERALS
Rich in calcium, magnesium, phosphorus, potassium, sodium, small amounts of copper and iron.

CALORIES PER 100G
38

Raspberry

Refreshing berry taste from dark pink juice. Goes well with peach, nectarine, apricot, apple.

PREPARATION
None – simply rinse.

VITAMINS
Rich in beta-carotene, biotin, C, small amounts of B1, B2, B3, B5, B6, E.

MINERALS
Rich in calcium, chlorine, magnesium, phosphorus, potassium, sulphur, sodium, iron, small amount of copper.

CALORIES PER 100G
25

Strawberry

The most vivid pink juice you've ever seen, a queen among juices with a taste that transports you into strawberry fields.

PREPARATION

None – remove green stalks if preferred.

VITAMINS

Rich in beta-carotene, folic acid, biotin, C, small amounts of B1, B2, B3, B5, B6, E.

MINERALS

Rich in calcium, chlorine, magnesium, phosphorus, potassium, sodium, sulphur, small amounts of copper, iron and zinc.

CALORIES PER 100G

26

Tangerine

Not so tart as orange, pale orange colour juice, slips down a treat on its own.

PREPARATION

Peel, chop into chunks.

VITAMINS

Rich in beta-carotene, folic acid, C, small amounts of B1, B2, B3, B5, B6.

MINERALS

Rich in calcium, magnesium, phosphorus, potassium, sodium, small amounts of copper, iron and manganese.

CALORIES PER 100G

35

Watermelon

A brownish/pink juice if you just use the flesh, but much darker if you juice the rind too, which increases the nutritional benefits. Very refreshing over the summer months.

Cut into quarters, do not remove pips, scoop flesh away from rind. if you're feeling adventurous you can use the rind too.

VITAMINS
Rich in beta-carotene, folic acid, B5, C, small amounts of B1, B2, B3, B6.

MINERALS
Rich in calcium, magnesium, phosphorus, potassium, sodium, small amounts of copper, iron and zinc.

CALORIES PER 100G
21

VEGETABLES

Alfalfa
A nutty-tasting juice, best used with other milder juices.

PREPARATION
None – simply rinse.

VITAMINS
Rich in beta-carotene, C, small amounts of B1, B2, B3.

MINERALS
Rich in calcium, phosphorus, potassium and sodium.

CALORIES PER 100G
30

Beansprout

Unappetizing looking, but full of useful nutrients; tastes better with sweeter juices.

PREPARATION

None – simply rinse.

VITAMINS

Rich in beta-carotene, C, small amounts of B1, B2, B3.

MINERALS

Rich in calcium, phosphorus, potassium, sodium, small amount of iron.

CALORIES PER 100G

29

Beetroot

This is a very potent purple juice – always mix it with other juices in a ratio of one part beetroot to four parts other juice.

PREPARATION

Cut off knobbly ends, scrub and chop into chunks.

VITAMINS

Rich in folic acid, C, small amounts of B1, B2, B3, B5.

MINERALS

Rich in calcium, magnesium, phosphorus, potassium, sodium, small amounts of copper, iron and zinc.

CALORIES PER 100G

44

Broccoli

A dark green juice, with a slightly bitter taste, should always be diluted with other milder juices by four parts to one.

PREPARATION
Cut into small florets, do not remove stalk.

VITAMINS
Rich in beta-carotene, folic acid, C, small amounts of B1, B2, B3, B5 and B6.

MINERALS
Rich in calcium, magnesium, phosphorus, potassium, sodium, small amounts of copper, iron and zinc.

CALORIES PER 100G
28

Brussels Sprout

Another strong dark green juice, which should always be diluted with a milder juice by four parts to one. It has a slightly bitter taste so combines well with sweeter juices such as carrot or apple.

PREPARATION
Remove dog-eared outer leaves, do not chop up.

VITAMINS
Rich in beta-carotene, folic acid, C, small amounts of B1, B2, B3, B5, B6.

MINERALS
Calcium, magnesium, phosphorus, potassium, sodium, small amounts of zinc, iron and copper.

CALORIES PER 100G
26

Cabbage (Red)

This juice has a wonderful dark purple colour and a slightly peppery taste. Like beetroot, it should be diluted with other milder juices four parts to one.

PREPARATION

Remove damaged outer leaves, cut into small chunks.

VITAMINS

Beta-carotene, folic acid, C, small amounts of B1, B2, B3, B5, B6.

MINERALS

Calcium, magnesium, phosphorus, potassium, sodium, small amounts of copper, iron and zinc.

CALORIES PER 100G

27

Cabbage (Winter)

This juice has a sulphurous smell and taste – better mixed with sweeter juices such as red pepper, parsnip or apple.

PREPARATION

Remove damaged outer leaves, cut into small chunks.

VITAMINS

Rich in beta-carotene, folic acid, C, small amounts of B1, B2, B3, B5, B6, biotin and E.

MINERALS

Rich in calcium, chlorine, magnesium, phosphorus, potassium, sodium, small amounts of copper, iron and zinc.

Cabbage (White)

A lovely sweet taste comes from this pale green juice.

PREPARATION

Remove damaged outer leaves, chop into small chunks.

VITAMINS

Rich in folic acid, C, small amounts of B1, B2, B3, B5, B6, biotin and E.

MINERALS

Calcium, chlorine, magnesium, phosphorus, potassium, sodium, small amounts of copper, iron and zinc.

CALORIES PER 100G

22

Carrot

This juice is ideal for mixing with all the other more potent juices. Its sweet but mild taste is great on its own too. It is the only vegetable juice that can be mixed with any fruit without anti-social consequences.

PREPARATION

Scrub, remove stalk end, chop into chunky strips.

VITAMINS

Rich in beta-carotene, folic acid, C, small amounts of B1, B2, B3, B5, B6, biotin and E.

MINERALS

Calcium, chlorine, magnesium, phosphorus, potassium, sodium, sulphur, small amounts of copper, iron and zinc.

CALORIES PER 100G
35

Cauliflower

A pale green juice, with a crisp, fresh aroma, good with sweeter juices.

PREPARATION
Cut into small florets, do not remove stalk.

VITAMINS
Rich in beta-carotene, folic acid, C, small amounts of B1, B2, B3, B5, B6.

MINERALS
Calcium, magnesium, phosphorus, potassium, sodium, small amounts of copper, iron and zinc.

CALORIES PER 100G
24

Celeriac

This light yellow juice tastes quite similar to celery, with a salty, refreshing flavour.
A good mixer.

PREPARATION
Rinse and chop into chunks.

VITAMINS
Rich in C, small amounts of B1, B2, B3, B6.

MINERALS
Rich in calcium, magnesium, phosphorus, potassium, sodium, small amount of iron.

18

Celery

This is a mild, salty-tasting juice, very good for mixing with more potent juices.

PREPARATION

Rinse and cut off bushy leaves.

VITAMINS

Rich in folic acid, C, small amounts of B1, B2, B3, B5, B6, biotin and E.

MINERALS

Rich in calcium, chlorine, manganese, phosphorus, potassium, sodium and sulphur.

CALORIES PER 100G

8

Cucumber

A watery, refreshing juice that goes very well with more potent varieties.

PREPARATION

Scrub outer skin (peel if you think it's waxed), cut into chunky strips.

VITAMINS

Rich in folic acid, C, small amounts of B1, B2, B3, B5, B6 and biotin.

MINERALS

Calcium, chlorine, magnesium, potassium, sodium, sulphur, small amounts of copper, iron and zinc.

CALORIES PER 100G

10

Fennel

If you love Pernod, you'll love fennel juice. Has a strong aniseed flavour – good for perking up blander juices.

PREPARATION
Slice bulb then chop into chunks.

VITAMINS
Rich in C, small amount of B6.

MINERALS
Calcium, potassium.

CALORIES PER 100G
28

Garlic

Adds excellent flavour – if you like garlic! But you only need a little, one or two cloves per glass of juice.

PREPARATION
Remove outer skin, chop and juice at the same time as a more sturdy vegetable.

VITAMINS
Rich in folic acid, C, small amounts of B1, B2, B3.

MINERALS
Rich in calcium, iron, magnesium, potassium, sodium, small amount of zinc.

CALORIES PER 100G
117

Kale

A strong dark green juice that should always be diluted by four parts to one with another milder juice.

PREPARATION
Remove damaged leaves, chop remaining kale into chunks.

VITAMINS
Rich in beta-carotene, B3, C, small amounts of B1, B2.

MINERALS
Calcium, iron, phosphorus, potassium and sodium.

CALORIES PER 100G
53

Leek

A light green juice with a pleasant oniony flavour, good for livening up a bland juice.

PREPARATION
Remove earthy stalk, cut into chunks widthways.

VITAMINS
Rich in beta-carotene, biotin, C, small amounts of B1, B2, B3, B5, B6, E.

MINERALS
Rich in calcium, chlorine, magnesium, phosphorus, potassium, sodium, small amounts of copper, iron and zinc.

CALORIES PER 100G
31

Lettuce

Lettuce is a dark green juice which should always be diluted by four parts to one with milder juice. It has quite a bitter taste, so needs to combine with a sweeter juice. You can choose from iceberg, round, and cos (which has the most nutrients). For convenience buy bags of ready rinsed salad leaves; oakleaf and lamb's lettuce are particularly tasty.

PREPARATION
Remove damaged leaves, chop into chunks.

VITAMINS
Rich in beta-carotene, C, small amounts of B1, B2, B3, B5, B6, E.

MINERALS
Rich in calcium, magnesium, phosphorus, potassium, sodium, small amounts of copper, iron and zinc.

CALORIES PER 100G
12–17

Mangetout (Snow Pea)

Bright green and sweet to the taste, dilute with a milder juice.

PREPARATION
None – simply rinse.

VITAMINS
Rich in beta-carotene, C, small amounts of B1, B2, B3.

MINERALS
Rich in calcium, iron, magnesium, phosphorus, potassium and sodium.

CALORIES PER 100G
42

Onion

Not for the faint-hearted! Creamy-coloured juice with a strong flavour. Best as a mixer.

PREPARATION
Peel, cut into chunks.

VITAMINS
Rich in folic acid, C, small amounts of B1, B2, B3, B5, B6, biotin.

MINERALS
Rich in calcium, chlorine, magnesium, phosphorus, potassium, sodium, sulphur, small amounts of copper, iron and zinc.

CALORIES PER 100G
23

Parsley

A strong green juice which should always be diluted by four parts to one. Nevertheless, a nice herby taste.

PREPARATION
Chop up and feed into juicer along with a more substantial vegetable.

VITAMINS
Rich in beta-carotene, B3, C, small amounts of B1, B2.

MINERALS
Rich in calcium, iron, phosphorus, potassium and sodium.

Parsnip

Don't turn your nose up – this juice has a deliciously sweet and creamy taste.

PREPARATION
Chop off earthy stalk, scrub and chop into chunks.

VITAMINS
Rich in folic acid, C, small amounts of B1, B2, B3, B5, B6, biotin and E.

MINERALS
Rich in calcium, chlorine, magnesium, phosphorus, potassium, sodium, sulphur, small amounts of copper, iron and zinc.

CALORIES PER 100G
49

Pepper (Bell – Red, Yellow and Green)

Pepper juice is delicious whether yellow, green or red, although red is sweeter and goes better with the more bitter juices.

PREPARATION
Chop into chunks.

VITAMINS
Rich in beta-carotene, folic acid, C, small amounts of B2, B3, B5 and B6, E.

MINERALS
Rich in calcium, chlorine, magnesium, phosphorus, potassium, sodium, small amounts of copper, iron and zinc.

Red, 32; Yellow, 26; Green, 15

Potato

A pale juice which doesn't taste particularly nice — better mixed in with something sweeter like carrot or parsnip.

PREPARATION

Scrub skin (only peel if very dirty), chop into chunks.

VITAMINS

Rich in folic acid, C, small amounts B1, B2, B3, B5, B6.

MINERALS

Calcium, chlorine, magnesium, phosphorus, potassium, sulphur, small amounts of copper, iron and zinc.

CALORIES PER 100G

87

Radish

Pink colour, peppery flavour, goes well with blander juices with which it should be diluted.

PREPARATION

None — simply rinse.

VITAMINS

Rich in folic acid, C, small amounts of B1, B2, B3, B5 and B6.

MINERALS

Rich in calcium, chlorine, iron, magnesium, phosphorus, potassium, sodium, sulphur, small amounts of copper and zinc.

CALORIES PER 100G
12

Spinach

Another dark green juice that must be diluted, four parts to one. Don't drink too much of it as it contains a substance called oxalic acid which can stop calcium from being absorbed.

PREPARATION

Rinse leaves, place in juicer with other more substantial vegetables (eg carrot, cucumber). Bags of baby leaf spinach are a useful stand by.

VITAMINS

Rich in beta-carotene, B3, C, small amounts of B1, B2.

MINERALS

Rich in calcium, iron, phosphorus, potassium and sodium.

CALORIES PER 100G
25

Sweet Potato

This juice has a similar taste to potato, but not quite so unappealing. It's a nice red/orange colour anyway!

PREPARATION

Scrub, chop into chunks.

VITAMINS

Rich in beta-carotene, folic acid, C, E, small amounts of B1, B2, B3, B5, B6.

Calcium, chlorine, magnesium, phosphorus, potassium, sodium, sulphur, small amounts of copper and iron.

CALORIES PER 100G
91

Tomato

Real tomato juice has a pinky/orange hue, and tastes like fresh tomatoes, not tomato paste. Excellent as a mixer, or drunk on its own.

PREPARATION
Rinse and chop into chunks. Do not peel.

VITAMINS
Rich in beta-carotene, biotin, folic acid, C, small amounts of B1, B2, B3, B5, B6.

MINERALS
Rich in chlorine, calcium, magnesium, phosphorus, potassium, sodium, sulphur, small amounts of copper, iron and zinc.

CALORIES PER 100G
14

Turnip

A bland-looking juice with a really peppery taste. Excellent for mixing with sweeter juices.

PREPARATION
Remove earthy stalk, scrub and cut into chunks.

VITAMINS
Rich in folic acid, C, small amounts of B1, B2, B3, B5, B6.

Rich in calcium, magnesium, phosphorus and potassium.

CALORIES PER 100G
20

Watercress

A strong green juice that must be diluted by four parts to one with other milder juices. Adds a nice, spicy taste.

PREPARATION
Rinse leaves, do not chop.

VITAMINS
Rich in beta-carotene, C, E, small amounts of B1, B2, B3, B5, B6, biotin.

MINERALS
Calcium, chlorine, iron, magnesium, phosphorus, potassium, sodium, sulphur, small amounts of copper and zinc.

CALORIES PER 100G
14

Wheatgrass

An acquired taste, wheatgrass juice is extremely potent, both in flavour and effect. It has a sweet, almost nauseating taste, yet with bitter undertones. Drink singly only in small (1–2 fl oz) servings; it tastes most palatable combined with apple or carrot juice. High in chlorophyll, wheatgrass is both cleansing and tonifying to the blood and organs.

PREPARATION
Wheatgrass is a somewhat specialised juice, usually available at juice bars, but is actually easy to grow at home. All you need is a packet of wheat grains (available from

wholefood/health food stores) and a shallow tray filled with about one inch of potting compost. Soak a cupful of grains in water overnight, then leave to drain during the day. That evening spread the grains in the tray, cover and leave for three days. After this time has elapsed, remove the cover, spray the grains with water, and place in a sunny spot for another three to four days (spraying with water each day). When the blades of wheatgerm are three or four inches high, they are ready to harvest. Cut a handful, rinse and juice. If you're using a high-street brand, non-specialist juicer, you may find it difficult to juice wheatgrass on its own. Instead, bunch up the wheatgrass and run it through the juicer with chunks of apple or carrot.

VITAMINS
Rich in beta-carotene, vitamin B complex, C and E.

MINERALS
Rich in calcium, iron, magnesium and potassium. Also contains enzymes to help digestion.

CALORIES PER 100G
Not applicable.

beauty, peak health and vitality

Incorporating freshly made juices into your diet is a simple way to enhance beauty, health and general wellbeing. They are packed with so many useful vitamins, minerals and other nutrients that it seems a shame not to benefit from their natural bounty. Chapters 4–6 focus on specific roles that juices can play, from improving your complexion to soothing sore throats, helping to calm nerves and combating insomnia. Among the juice recipes you will find vegetable and fruit juice combinations – don't just stick to one type, vary them to get maximum benefit: for example, a vegetable-based juice in the morning, a fruit one in the evening, or vegetable juices one day, fruit the next.

Children

The juice recommendations given are for adults and do not apply to children. As a guideline, children younger than thirteen should not drink more than 5 fl oz/145ml of raw juice a day, and should always drink their juice diluted with water. Teenagers can begin to drink undiluted juices, but no more than one to two servings per day. Dilution is necessary because fresh juices can be rather thick in consistency and strong in taste, are always very concentrated, and may be too potent for young digestive systems.

Adults

Adult digestive systems can cope better with undiluted juice, but many of us find that we prefer to drink juices diluted too. As a general rule, unless you are very used to drinking raw fruit and vegetable juices, don't drink more than three 8 fl oz/230ml glasses of juice a day. And do remember to vary your intake, so that you benefit from a broad spectrum of nutrients.

Extras

You can zip up any of these juices with additions like fresh herbs (such as coriander, mint, oregano, marjoram and basil) and fresh and ground spices (such as ginger, nutmeg, cinnamon, allspice and liquorice sticks). You can also add honey for extra sweetness, wheatgerm (an excellent source of vitamin E and the B complex group of vitamins), plain live yoghurt (excellent for the digestive system), or semi-skimmed milk to turn them into milk shakes. For extra energy you can blend in some mashed banana or avocado, both high in minerals, particularly potassium. See Chapter 8 for more ideas on how to liven up juices.

Remember these general guidelines:

- Juicing novices can drink up to three 8 fl oz/230ml glasses of juice a day, but veterans can drink up to six (their bodies will be more used to the potent effects of juice).
- Avoid mixing vegetable and fruit juices, or you may experience uncomfortable flatulence or bloating. The exceptions are apple and carrot.
- Vary your juice intake throughout the week. In particular, don't overdo the strong green juices (such as spinach and watercress) or the citrus juices which have a very strong cleansing effect. Stick to one 8 fl oz/230ml glass of these juices three to four times a week.
- Stick to vegetable rather than fruit juices if you suffer from diabetes, low blood sugar or candidiasis (see page 107).
- If you want to alter any of the recipes to suit your own tastes, remember that carrot and apple juices are very good mixers and can make an unappealing combination more palatable.

juices for beauty

Do you long for a clear complexion? Bright eyes? Lustrous, shiny hair? Strong, healthy nails? It's not an impossible dream. The condition of our external features is not just determined by our genes and the weather, it can be greatly influenced by what we eat and drink too. Foods rich in nutrients like vitamins A, C, E and beta-carotene, and the minerals zinc and potassium, are the key to a more beautiful you.

EYES

Like every other part of our body, eyes should not be taken for granted. They work hard every day, and have to deal with pollution, bits of dust, even fragments of makeup falling into them. A plentiful supply of the 'eye' vitamins, B complex, C, E and beta-carotene, won't enable you to see in the dark, but they will help to keep eyes clear and bright.

Juices

Each recipe makes approx. 8 fl oz/230ml glass of juice. Adults can drink up to three glasses daily, but do vary the juice combinations for maximum benefit (for children see page 49). Dilute with water if you prefer. Juice each ingredient then blend using a spoon.

2 large carrots
4 broccoli florets
4 cauliflower florets

or

3 tomatoes
handful of watercress
½ red (bell) pepper

or

1 grapefruit
1 mango (I prefer organic mangoes, they seem to be riper and more juicy)
1 passion fruit

or

4 tangerines
1 pear

HEALTHY HAIR

Hair is our crowning glory – why not endeavour to make it look as good as possible?
Hair that has been dyed or permed can look dull and lifeless, but so too can totally
natural hair that is lacking vital nutrients. The external hair shaft is actually dead, but
the root is alive and is fed essential minerals and vitamins through the bloodstream.

High Gloss

Vitamins from the B complex group, and the minerals iron, iodine and sulphur, are
essential for healthy hair and can be supplied by a range of fresh juices.

Juices

Each recipe makes approx. one 8 fl oz/230ml glass of juice. Adults can drink up to three
glasses daily, but do vary the juice combinations for maximum benefit (for children see
page 49). Dilute with water if you prefer. Juice each ingredient then blend using a spoon.

4oz/125g chunk winter cabbage

2 large carrots

6 radishes

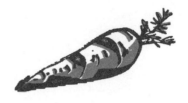

or

4oz/125g mangetout (snow peas)

3 kale leaves

2 large carrots

½ parsnip

or

4 tangerines

4oz/125g raspberries

or

small bunch grapes

2 passion fruit

2 thick slices pineapple

Anti-Dandruff

Dandruff can occur for two reasons: either the sebaceous glands in the scalp do not produce enough lubricating oil (sebum), or they produce too much. In the first case, skin flakes off, and hair goes dry and brittle; in the second the dandruff is yellow and the hair greasy. Juices rich in the B group of vitamins, vitamin E, and beta-carotene may help improve the condition of your scalp.

Juices

Each recipe makes approx. one 8 fl oz/230ml glass of juice. Adults can drink up to three glasses daily, but do vary the juice combinations for maximum benefit (for children see page 49). Dilute with water if you prefer. Juice each ingredient then blend using a spoon.

2½ large carrots
6 kale leaves

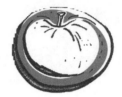

or

½ lettuce
2 small apples

or

1 mango (I prefer organic mangoes, they seem to be riper and more juicy)
1 peach
1 apple

or

small bunch of grapes
2 kiwi fruit

NAILS

Like hair, nails are dead once they emerge from the cuticle, but as they grow beneath the skin of the finger, they can display visible signs that we may be short of certain nutrients, particularly minerals. White spots on the nails may represent a need for more zinc, and brittle nails often indicate lack of iron. The trace minerals, sulphur and iodine, and vitamin B2 (riboflavin) are also important for the growth of strong, healthy nails.

Juices

Each recipe makes approx. one 8 fl oz/230ml glass of juice. Adults can drink up to three glasses daily, but do vary the juice combinations for maximum benefit (for children see page 49). Dilute with water if you prefer. Juice each ingredient then blend using a spoon.

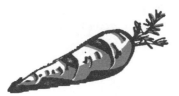

4oz/125g beansprouts
4oz/125g chunk white cabbage
2 large carrots

or

¼ cucumber
4oz/125g Brussels sprouts
3 tomatoes

or

4oz/125g blackberries
4oz/125g strawberries
1 apple

or

1 orange
3 apricots

SKIN

The skin is particularly affected by sluggish digestion and overworked kidneys. If your kidneys can't cope with the amount of waste being generated by your daily intake of food and drink, the toxins will come out via your skin instead, sometimes causing blemishes to appear.

Fresh fruit and vegetable juices can help detoxify your body and stimulate the kidneys (see Chapter 7 for a full detox plan), and a whole range of juices can feed the skin with much-needed vitamins and minerals.

The onset of lines and wrinkles might be delayed a little with a regular intake of juices containing the antioxidant nutrients: vitamins A, C, E, beta-carotene and the mineral selenium. These have the ability to quench the unstable molecules called free radicals which play a role in the ageing process. Try the juice recipes below for a range of skin problems.

Super Skin

To keep skin looking clear of blemishes, well-toned and healthy, you need juices that are high in vitamins C, E and beta-carotene, the minerals zinc and potassium, together with juices that stimulate the digestive system and kidneys to work efficiently, such as beetroot, parsley and spinach.

Juices

Each recipe makes approx. one 8 fl oz/230ml glass of juice. Adults can drink up to three glasses daily, but do vary the juice combinations for maximum benefit (for children see page 49). Dilute with water if you prefer. Juice each ingredient then blend using a spoon.

¼ red (bell) pepper
¼ green (bell) pepper
⅓ large cucumber

or

¼ head fennel
2oz/50g chunk red cabbage
1½ apples

or

2 large carrots
2 stalks celery
small bunch parsley

or

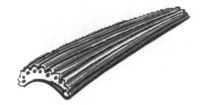

1 large orange
5oz/150g strawberries
2oz/50g blueberries

or

3oz/75g cranberries
1½ apples

Wrinkle-Buster

The existence of an elixir of eternal life and youth remains in the realms of myth, but scientists have recently discovered that everyday vitamins and minerals may combat premature ageing. The antioxidants beta-carotene, vitamins C, E, and the mineral selenium are thought to help delay the onset of lines and wrinkles (see page 5). These nutrients also feed collagen, the vital substance that keeps skin elastic and flexible.

Juices

Each recipe makes approx. one 8 fl oz/230ml glass of juice. Adults can drink up to three glasses daily, but do vary the juice combinations for maximum benefit. Dilute with water if you prefer. Juice each ingredient then blend using a spoon.

3 large carrots
2oz/50g parsley

or

4oz/125g chunk of kale
1 apple
1½ large carrots

or

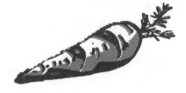

1 medium grapefruit
1 small orange

or

1 peach
5oz/150g raspberries
3 guavas

Acne

Whether acne strikes during teenage years, or continues into adult life, it is one of those conditions that is irritating and unsightly. Acne can be hereditary or caused by an imbalance of hormones. It causes the skin's sebum glands to produce too much grease, which then becomes infected by bacteria. The main sites are the back, shoulders, chest, neck and face. Juices rich in the nutrients beta-carotene and zinc can be of benefit to acne sufferers.

Juices

Each recipe makes approx. one 8 fl oz/230ml glass of juice. Adults can drink up to three glasses daily, but do vary the juice combinations for maximum benefit. Dilute with water if you prefer. Juice each ingredient then blend using a spoon.

2½ large carrots
4oz/125g watercress

or

3 tomatoes
8 small broccoli florets

or

1 apple
1 mango (I prefer organic mangoes, they seem to be riper and more juicy)
5oz/150g raspberries

or

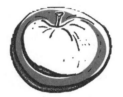

3 apricots
6oz/175g cherries
1 nectarine

juices for health

Fresh juices are not an instant cure for the numerous common complaints to which we may be prone at one time or another, but they can provide a bountiful supply of nutrients, to help increase our sapped strength and hasten recovery. Their cleansing power can also help in flushing toxins from the body; green, leafy vegetables, for example, are particularly rich in chlorophyll, which has been shown to have antiseptic properties and can build up red blood cells. And when you don't feel like eating, a glass of health-giving fresh juice may be just what you need.

BREATHE EASY

Every year, most of us will go down with a minor respiratory illness – it's almost guaranteed. It could be a cold, cough, sore throat, flu or bronchitis. Whichever bug we pick up, it's bound to make us feel miserable and lethargic for a couple of days at least. Inflamed throat, sore and chapped nose, high temperature, fatigue and loss of appetite are all inevitable results of a virulent bug – perhaps caught in a crowded train or at the office.

These disabling symptoms are not only restricted to the autumn and winter (although they are more prevalent at this time). Respiratory infections can occur in the spring and summer too, often at the changeover period between seasons, when your body is in flux as it acclimatizes itself to heat, or to cold, dry, or damp weather conditions.

Juices can soothe the throat, calm a tickly cough, and provide a nutritious energy boost. Juices can also help to ease a sore throat in the case of more persistent and semi-permanent conditions such as asthma, hay fever and allergic rhinitis.

Colds and Sore Throats

The common cold can be caused by one of 200 viruses and affects the mucous membranes of the nose and throat. The cold viruses are some of the most elusive bugs ever known and after 40 years of intense research by some of the world's top scientists there is still no cure or vaccination for that well-known set of symptoms – sneezing, tickly throat, cough, watering eyes and headache.

Like many other viruses, the cold bug is passed easily from one person to another in a crowded space. Once inside your body, it incubates for a day, before manifesting itself as a cold.

Vitamin C is the number one nutrient needed, as it increases resistance to infection. Citrus fruits are an excellent source of vitamin C and also have astringent properties which can tighten mucous membranes to make breathing easier. Also useful is a beta-carotene, which helps to protect and tonify the mucous membranes of the body; vitamin E which supports the work of beta-carotene; and zinc which may hasten your recovery from the cold. Garlic juice can also be very beneficial as it is strongly anti-viral (because it is so pungent, you only need a tiny amount, mixed in with other vegetable juices).

Juices

Each recipe makes approx. one 8 fl oz/230ml glass of juice. Adults can drink up to three glasses daily, but do vary the juice combinations for maximum benefit (for children see page 49). Dilute with water if you prefer. Juice each ingredient then blend using a spoon.

3 large carrots
2oz/50g parsley
2 cloves garlic

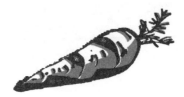

or

handful of watercress
¼ cucumber
4oz/125g chunk white cabbage
2 cloves garlic

or

2 kiwi fruit
½ mango (I prefer organic mangoes, they seem to be riper and more juicy)
1 medium apple

or

1 grapefruit
1 orange
4oz/125g strawberries

Coughs and Bronchitis

Coughs can range from a tickly irritation at the back of the throat to a full-blown chest infection with copious phlegm that is part of a nasty cold or even bronchitis. Coughing is generally the result of inflammation of the mucous membranes, either in the throat or in the bronchi (the tiny tubes that make up the inner lung).

One of the most useful purposes served by fresh juices in the case of a cough is their power to soothe. A glass of thick home-made juice can lubricate dried mucous membranes in the throat. Citrus juices have the special quality of acting as an astringent on the mucous membranes, which makes it easier to breathe. Juices rich in beta-carotene can also help protect the mucous membranes, and of course extra supplies of vitamin C are very useful. Onion juice is also an old naturopathic remedy for catarrh – it has a very strong flavour, but you could give it a try mixed with other beneficial juices, as in the recipe for carrot, onion and broccoli juice below.

Juices

Each recipe makes approx. one 8 fl oz/230ml glass of juice. Adults can drink up to three glasses daily, but do vary the juice combinations for maximum benefit (for children see page 49). Dilute with water if you prefer. Juice each ingredient then blend using a spoon.

2 large carrots
½ medium onion
4 broccoli florets

or

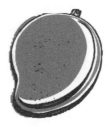

½ green (bell) pepper
4oz/125g chunk red cabbage
3 tomatoes
or

½ medium pineapple
½ mango (I prefer organic mangoes, they seem to be riper and more juicy)
3 plums

or

4 tangerines
½ lemon
1 tsp/5ml honey

Flu

Although you can contract flu in the summer, it is far more common in the winter, when strains move steadily around the globe. Flu is caused by a virus, but, as in the case of colds, it is not always the same one. That is why, although you may have had flu before, you can contract it again because your body has not built up an immunity to the new strain.

Symptoms of flu include sore throat, cough, runny nose, aches and pains, fever, fatigue and loss of appetite. A sore throat benefits from the soothing effects of juice, which also provides essential vitamin C and beta-carotene. Juices should be drunk diluted if you have flu and are not eating – this is because the high levels of natural sugar contained in fruits and some vegetables can make you feel a little dizzy if drunk on an empty stomach.

Juices

Each recipe makes approx. one 8 fl oz/230ml glass of juice. Adults can drink up to three glasses daily, but do vary the juice combinations for maximum benefit (for children see page 49). Dilute with water if you prefer. Juice each ingredient then blend using a spoon.

2 large carrots
½ leek
2oz/50g parsley

or

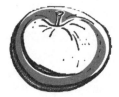

2oz/50g Brussels sprouts
2 tomatoes
¼ cucumber

or

4 tangerines
1 papaya

or

small bunch of grapes
2 kiwi-fruit
1 apple

Asthma, Hay Fever and Allergic Rhinitis

These are all conditions which are triggered by certain situations. In the case of asthma it can be over-exertion, anxiety, smoke, cold or some other external cause. Hay fever is provoked by tree, grass and flower pollens, and allergic rhinitis can be caused by anything from dust to chemicals to cat dander. Juices can help soothe coughing, and build up the body's reserve of nutrients used in immunity, such as vitamin C, beta-carotene, the B complex group of vitamins, and the mineral zinc. As stress can also provoke or heighten these conditions, the B vitamins may help to calm you down.

Juices

Each recipe makes approx. one 8 fl oz/230ml glass of juice. Adults can drink up to three glasses daily, but do vary the juice combinations for maximum benefit (for children see page 49). Dilute with water if you prefer. Juice each ingredient then blend using a spoon.

¼ lettuce
2 tomatoes
2 large carrots

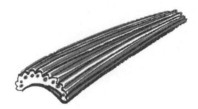

or

8 broccoli florets
3 celery stalks

or

4oz/125g raspberries
4oz/125g strawberries
1 orange

or

1 peach
1 nectarine
8 cherries

BURNS AND SCALDS

Minor burns are a common hazard in the home. As soon as one has occurred you should hold the affected part of your body under the cold tap for several minutes; this helps the skin to cool down, and restricts the area affected by the burn. Drinking juices rich in vitamin C and E may also help speed recovery afterwards.

Juices

Each recipe makes approx. one 8 fl oz/230ml glass of juice. Adults can drink up to three glasses daily, but do vary the juice combinations for maximum benefit (for children see page 49). Dilute with water if you prefer. Juice each ingredient then blend using a spoon.

4oz/125g blackcurrants
4oz/125g raspberries
1 peach

or

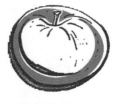

1 grapefruit
1 kiwi fruit
½ lime

or

¼ medium sweet potato
4 tomatoes
¼ medium lettuce

or

1 apple
2oz parsley
¼ large cucumber

CRAMP

Cramps are involuntary muscle spasms that usually occur in the calves or feet. It can occasionally be due to lack of body salt or bad circulation, but continuous use of certain muscles, such as during exercise workouts, and long periods spent in one position are more common causes. Usual nutrients are sodium (if you eat very little processed food or salt, or sweat a lot) and the mineral magnesium.

Sodium Loss

Juices

Each recipe makes approx. one 8 fl oz/230ml glass of juice. Adults can drink up to three glasses daily, but do vary the juice combinations for maximum benefit (for children see page 49). Dilute with water if you prefer. Juice each ingredient then blend using a spoon.

3 stalks celery
¼ cucumber

or

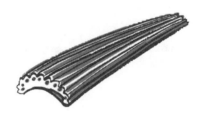

½ head celeriac
2 large carrots

or

5oz/150g cherries
1 apple

or

1 medium melon

Lack of magnesium

Juices

Each recipe makes approx. one 8 fl oz/230ml glass of juice. Adults can drink up to three glasses daily, but do vary the juice combinations for maximum benefit (for children see page 49). Dilute with water if you prefer. Juice each ingredient then blend using a spoon.

2 passion fruit
8oz/225g grapes

or

8oz/225g strawberries
2 guavas

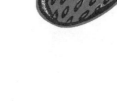

or

4oz/125g mangetout (snow peas)
½ parsnip
2 large carrots

or

¼ beetroot
½ head celeriac
¼ large cucumber

DIGESTION

Indigestion, constipation and bad breath are among the most common and frequent ailments to beset us. It's hardly surprising when you consider how busily the digestive system works all day long, supplied with almost constant food and drink. The meals that we eat are often too late, too much, too quick, too spicy, too fatty, and low in fibre; our chosen drinks are often fizzy, or caffeine-based; none of which helps our digestive systems to function at their best.

In addition to including more wholefoods and fibre-rich fruit and vegetables in your diet, fresh juices can help to keep the digestive organs healthy and well-toned. Better digestion means that more nutrients will be absorbed too.

Juices that help nourish this area of the body are rich in the B group of vitamins, vitamin C, beta-carotene and the mineral chlorine.

Bad Breath

Bad breath can be caused by a number of things, including indigestion, constipation, illness, lack of food, dental decay, gum disease and too much rich or spicy food. As well as eating plenty of fibre-rich wholefoods to help the digestive process, some juices can help to freshen breath, especially parsley and carrot. Try these combinations.

Juices

Each recipe makes approx. one 8 fl oz/230ml glass of juice. Adults can drink up to three glasses daily, but do vary the juice combinations for maximum benefit (for children see page 49). Dilute with water if you prefer. Juice each ingredient then blend using a spoon.

4oz/115g parsley
3 large carrots

or

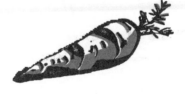

1 apple
2 stalks celery
2oz/50g parsley

Indigestion

One of the commonest complaints around, indigestion is easy to set right. The causes are usually simple, for example over-eating, eating too fast, eating the wrong kinds of food, heavy smoking and anxiety. Certain juices make excellent *digestifs*.

Pineapple juice contains bromelain, an enzyme which can help balance the levels of acidity and alkalinity in the system; and papaya juice contains an enzyme called papain which can break down protein, and therefore help your own stomach enzymes to digest food. Garlic juice can also help soothe the gut.

Juices

Each recipe makes approx. one 8 fl oz/230ml glass of juice. Adults can drink up to three glasses daily, but do vary the juice combinations for maximum benefit (for children see page 49). Dilute with water if you prefer. Juice each ingredient then blend using a spoon.

½ papaya
4fl oz/115ml still water

or

½ papaya
½ peach
2fl oz/50ml still water

or

2 thick slices pineapple
1 mango (I prefer organic mangoes, they seem to be riper and more juicy)

or

3 tomatoes
1 clove garlic
1 stalk celery

or

3 large carrots
1 clove garlic

Constipation

Constipation is usually the result of a diet low in fibre and high in processed foods.
It can cause headaches, fatigue, bad breath and poor skin. Although many people go
without passing a stool for several days, it really is best for your body to have a bowel
movement at least once a day, so that toxins are not sitting around for too long. In peak
bowel health, it takes about 8-12 hours for food to be fully digested, nutrients absorbed
and for waste to be passed out.

Fibre-rich foods, such as raw fruit and vegetables, brown bread and wholegrains, can
make an enormous difference to your regularity, but so too can juices, even though they
do not contain much fibre. All fresh juices have an excellent cleansing effect on the gut
and bowel and have a gentle laxative effect. The dark green juices, such as kale, spinach
and watercress can be particularly useful (they are rich in minerals and the B complex
group of vitamins), as can the fruit juices pear, papaya, grape and watermelon (which all
have a cleansing effect).

Juices

Each recipe makes approx. one 8 fl oz/230ml glass of juice. Adults can drink up to three
glasses daily, but do vary the juice combinations for maximum benefit (for children see
page 49). Dilute with water if you prefer. Juice each ingredient then blend using a
spoon.

6 large spinach leaves
4 tomatoes
1 chunk cucumber

or

2 large carrots
handful of watercress
½ apple

or

1 pear
5oz/150g grapes

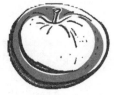

or

½ medium watermelon
4fl oz/115ml still water

Diarrhoea

Food poisoning, stress and viruses can all cause diarrhoea, which can also go hand in hand with uncomfortable stomach gripes. Anyone suffering from it should drink plenty of liquids, including some mild fresh juices, diluted with water. Varieties that can help settle a disturbed digestive system are apple, carrot and pineapple, best drunk on their own and diluted.

Juices

Each recipe makes approx. one 8 fl oz/230ml glass of juice. Adults can drink up to three glasses daily, but do vary the juice combinations for maximum benefit (for children see page 49). Dilute with water if you prefer. Juice each ingredient then blend using a spoon.

1 apple
4fl oz/115ml still water

or

2 large carrots
4fl oz/115ml still water

or

2 thick slices pineapple
4fl oz/115ml still water

Irritable Bowel Syndrome

Diarrhoea interspersed with constipation are the classic symptoms of irritable bowel syndrome, which can be brought on by stress, as well as other causes. Mild, yet nutritious juices (containing B vitamins and vitamin C) may help settle the stomach and bring a little relief. It is best not to overwhelm the stomach with combination juices, and the juices should be diluted before drinking.

Juices

Each recipe makes approx. one 8 fl oz/230ml glass of juice. Adults can drink up to three glasses, diluted, daily, but do vary the juices for maximum benefit. Juice each ingredient then blend using a spoon.

1 apple
4fl oz/115ml still water

or

1 pear
4fl oz/115ml still water

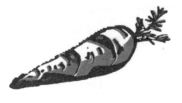

or

1½ carrots
4fl oz/115ml still water

or

2 stalks celery
4fl oz/115ml still water

Nausea and Vomiting

These conditions can have a variety of causes. It could be an infectious bug, such as food poisoning, too much alcohol, too much fatty food, morning sickness during pregnancy, or travel sickness. A mild juice high in vitamin C and the B complex group of vitamins may help speed recovery and quell feelings of nausea. Fennel juice with its aniseed taste can also calm a queasy tummy. Add a teaspoon of ground ginger (preferably fresh) to add to the benefits.

Dilute the juice, so that no extra strain is placed on your stomach.

Juices

Each recipe makes approx. one 8 fl oz/230ml glass of juice. Adults can drink up to three glasses, diluted, daily, but do vary the juices for maximum benefit (for children see page 49). Juice each ingredient then blend using a spoon.

1 grapefruit
fresh ground ginger
4fl oz/115ml still water

or

½ melon
fresh ground ginger
4fl oz/115ml still water

or

1 orange
fresh ground ginger
4fl oz/115ml still water

or

½ head fennel
fresh ground ginger
4fl oz/115ml still water

OVERWEIGHT

Gone are the days when the perfect figure was considered that of a stick insect, but
there are still important health reasons why you should not let your body become
overweight. It puts greater strain on the heart, lungs and joints, increasing the risk of
heart disease, high blood pressure, varicose veins, diabetes and hernias.

   Opting for fresh fruit and vegetables, wholegrains, pulses, fish and lean meat, instead
of processed foods and foods high in saturated fat, can help you to lose extra pounds.
Naturally, low-calorie fresh juices can play a useful role too, and are excellent
replacement snacks.

Juices

Each recipe makes approx. one 8 fl oz/230ml glass of juice. Adults can drink up to three
glasses daily, but do vary the juice combinations for maximum benefit (for children see
page 49). Dilute with water if you prefer. Juice each ingredient then blend using a
spoon.

4 oz/125g gooseberries
1 peach
1 passion fruit

or

3 apricots
4oz/125g blackberries
1 nectarine

or

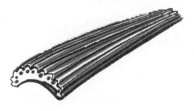

2 large carrots
4 broccoli florets
4oz/125g alfalfa sprouts

or

3 stalks celery
2 tomatoes
handful of watercress

RELIEF FROM ACHES AND PAINS

Conditions like rheumatism and arthritis can be crippling, but more often than not
produce regular nagging pain. It's the same story with gall stones, headaches and
migraine. Juices can't claim to cure any of these ailments, but they may help to alleviate
the symptoms.

Arthritis and Rheumatism

There are two types of arthritis – rheumatoid and osteo. In rheumatoid arthritis, wrists,
knuckles, knees and feet tend to become the most inflamed part of the body, whereas in
osteoarthritis, it is often the cartilage linings around weight-bearing joints such as hips
that degenerate, causing inflammation, pain and stiffness. Arthritis often occurs,
therefore, in areas of the body which take the greatest wear and tear during our
lifetimes. Rheumatism is an umbrella term for both types of arthritis, and also aches
and pains that often come on during damp and chilly weather.

Celery juice, with its high concentrations of sodium and potassium, is the vegetable juice most often recommended by naturopaths as an excellent natural remedy against both kinds of arthritis and rheumatism. Pineapple juice may also help because it contains bromelain (an enzyme which has anti-inflammatory properties).

Juices

Each recipe makes approx. one 8 fl oz/230ml glass of juice. Adults can drink up to two glasses daily, but do vary the juice combinations for maximum benefit (for children see page 49). Drink diluted with water if you prefer. Juice each ingredient then blend using a spoon.

3 stalks celery
¼ cucumber

or

3 stalks celery
1 carrot

or

2 stalks celery
1 apple

or

½ medium pineapple
1 mango (I prefer organic mangoes, they seem to be riper and more juicy)

Headaches and Migraines

Tension, the atmosphere (e.g. certain weather conditions, air conditioning and traffic pollution), food allergies, general illness and eyestrain can all cause headaches and in the worst cases migraine. Headaches range from sharp shooting pains to all-enveloping aches that can radiate down the neck. Celery juice can help to alleviate headache pains as it has a high sodium and potassium content. Juices rich in the B complex group of vitamins may also be useful.

Juices

Each recipe makes approx. one 8 fl oz/230ml glass of juice. Adults can drink up to three glasses daily, but do vary the juice combinations for maximum benefit (for children see page 49). Dilute with water if you prefer. Juice each ingredient then blend using a spoon.

¼ turnip
½ red (bell) pepper
2 large carrots

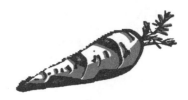

or

2oz/50g sweet potato
½ leek
3 stalks celery

or

3 tangerines
2 guavas

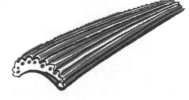

or

3 apricots
6oz/175g cherries

PROTECTING AGAINST DEGENERATIVE DISEASE

Research over the last few years has suggested that a diet high in fruit and vegetables may contribute to lowering the risk of developing degenerative diseases such as heart disease and some cancers. As a result of current thinking, the World Health Organisation has advised that we should be consuming at least 14oz/400g of fresh fruit and vegetables a day to maintain our health.

The following juices contain beta-carotene, vitamins C, E and selenium, and can be drunk on a regular basis to provide all-round goodness – but don't forget to keep eating whole fruit and vegetables too. See Chapter 8 for more healthy recipes.

Juices

Each recipe makes approx. one 8 fl oz/230ml glass of juice. Adults can drink up to three glasses daily, but do vary the juice combinations for maximum benefit (for children see page 49). Dilute with water if you prefer. Juice each ingredient then blend using a spoon.

2 large carrots
1 mango (I prefer organic mangoes, they seem to be riper and more juicy)

or

1 medium cantaloupe melon

or

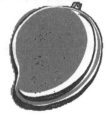

3 large carrots
6 large spinach leaves

or

1 nectarine
1 peach

or

¼ sweet potato
2 tomatoes
2 large carrots

or

handful of watercress
2 large carrots
¼ red (bell) pepper

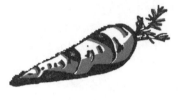

or

2 large carrots
8 small broccoli florets
1 chunk cucumber

WELL WOMAN

Today, more than ever, women need to look after their health. As life has become
steadily more pressurized, so the stresses and strains to which women are subjected
have increased. A woman may be working full-time and holding together a family –
cooking, cleaning, planning – being friend, mother and lover, all at once.

As the emphasis of health care moves increasingly towards prevention rather than
cure, women can use natural ways to alleviate some minor, yet irritating, conditions.
They can also take control of their diet and make sure that they are providing their
bodies with the best possible nutrition. Fresh juices, as well as other natural and
unprocessed foods, have a role to play in achieving this.

Anaemia

Anaemia (not the pernicious variety) is a common problem among women who do not absorb enough iron and folic acid through their diet. A lack of these nutrients affects the production of red blood cells (haemoglobin). It can also occur among those who have very heavy periods, through which too many red blood cells are lost.

Symptoms are pale skin, pale lining of the mouth, and sore tongue, often accompanied by fatigue and lack of energy. The following juices contain moderate levels of iron and folic acid, but if you are anaemic to some degree, it is wise to increase your intake of fish, red meat, liver and dried fruits too.

Juices

Each recipe makes approx. one 8 fl oz/230ml glass of juice. Adults can drink up to three glasses daily, but do vary the juice combinations for maximum benefit. Dilute with water if you prefer. Juice each ingredient then blend using a spoon.

4oz/125g chunk of red cabbage
2 large carrots
2oz/50g parsley

or

¼ beetroot
2oz/50g chunk kale
2½ large carrots

or

½ medium pineapple
2 passion fruit
1 tangerine

or

6oz/175g strawberries
2oz/50g blackberries
1 apple

Cystitis

Cystitis is an inflammation of the bladder usually caused by bacteria from the anus which finds its way into the urethra. It is a painful and uncomfortable condition, and seems to recur. Symptoms can include the urgent need to urinate while only a small amount of urine actually comes out; a painful, burning feeling when urinating; pain in the abdomen, buttocks and back; and urine streaked with blood, or pink in colour.

The best way to flush the infecting bacteria from the bladder is to drink plenty of water (adding a teaspoonful of bicarbonate of soda can help). Diluted fruit and vegetable juices can also help to flush out bacteria and create a more alkaline environment within the digestive tract and bladder. Cranberry juice and most other berry juices are very effective as they prevent bacteria from adhering to the mucous membrane of the bladder, and garlic juice is a natural antiseptic that can help cleanse the area.

Juices

Each recipe makes approx. one 8 fl oz/230ml glass of juice. Adults can drink up to three glasses, diluted, daily, but do vary the juice combinations for maximum benefit (for children see page 49). Juice each ingredient then blend using a spoon.

5oz/150g cranberries
6fl oz/170ml still water

or

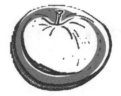

1 apple
1 pear
3fl oz/80ml still water

or

¼ cucumber
2 large carrots
2oz/50g parsley
2 cloves garlic

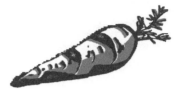

or

4oz/125g alfalfa sprouts
4 tomatoes
¼ green (bell) pepper

Premenstrual Syndrome

This syndrome recurs with each monthly cycle, and includes physical, mental and emotional symptoms. It is a common problem among women, between two and ten days before their periods. Typical PMS sufferers experience mood swings, depression, fluid retention, food cravings, skin blemishes and abdominal cramps. The probable cause of these symptoms is an imbalance of the female hormones progesterone and oestrogen. The B complex group of vitamins are thought to help, as are extra supplies of the minerals magnesium, potassium, zinc, iron and calcium.

Juices

Each recipe makes approx. one 8 fl oz/230ml glass of juice. Adults can drink up to three glasses daily (for girls see page 49), but do vary the juice combinations for maximum benefit. Dilute with water if you prefer. Juice each ingredient then blend using a spoon.

4oz/125g kale
2 large carrots
¼ red (bell) pepper

or

½ leek
¼ medium sweet potato
1 apple

or

½ pineapple
4oz/125g raspberries

or

2 kiwi fruit
2 guavas
1 pear

Pregnancy

It's a myth to say that pregnant women need to eat twice as much as usual, but they are wise to ensure that their diet is nutritionally rich and varied, for the health of their baby and themselves. As well as eating plenty of wholesome foods, expectant mothers can help top up supplies of essential vitamins and minerals by drinking a range of fresh juices. Pregnant women should dilute juices, so they are not too concentrated.

Juices

Each recipe makes approx. one 8 fl oz/230ml glass of juice. Drink up to three glasses diluted, daily, but do vary the juice combinations for maximum benefit. Juice each ingredient then blend using a spoon.

2 large carrots
1 apple

or

½ medium pineapple
1 mango (I prefer organic mangoes, they seem to be riper and more juicy)

or

2 large carrots
4oz/125g cauliflower
1 tomato

or

4 kale leaves
2 stalks celery
2 tomatoes

Menopause

Women going through the menopause experience physical change because they have come to an end of their childbearing years. Levels of the hormones oestrogen and progesterone drop significantly, and menstruation gradually declines.

For many women, a knock-on result of this can be osteoporosis (reduced density of the bones). This is because the presence of oestrogen helps to keep bones dense, and once supplies dwindle they become less solid. Extra calcium and magnesium are necessary to supplement the gap left by lack of oestrogen. Fresh juices are a good source of these two minerals, as are food sources such as milk, cheese, fish and nuts.

Juices

Each recipe makes approx. one 8 fl oz/230ml glass of juice. Drink up to three glasses daily, but do vary the juice combinations for maximum benefit. Dilute with water if you prefer. Juice each ingredient then blend using a spoon.

2 kiwi fruit

2 guavas

1 apple

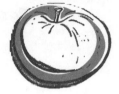

or

6oz/175g strawberries

1 grapefruit

or

3 large carrots

6 kale leaves

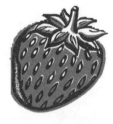

or

¼ medium turnip

3 tomatoes

1 stalk celery

Water Retention

Water retention often occurs around period time, as a result of the changing hormone balance in a woman's body. There are several juices which act as diuretics (substances which help eliminate excess fluid through the flow of urine). The best of these are celery, cucumber, cranberry, strawberry and watermelon; all are moderately high in minerals, such as potassium and sodium.

Juices

Each recipe makes approx. one 8 fl oz/230ml glass of juice. Adults can drink up to three glasses daily, but do vary the juice combinations for maximum benefit. Dilute with water if you prefer. Juice each ingredient then blend using a spoon.

2 large carrots
3 stalks celery

or

¼ large cucumber
¼ parsnip
2oz/50g parsley

or

1½ apples
5oz/150g cranberries

or

1 small watermelon

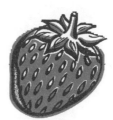

or

6oz/175g strawberries
2 thick slices pineapple

WOUND HEALING

Wounds can be external cuts and abrasions or inner disruptions caused by operations, tears, and other injuries. Juices high in vitamins C, E, the B complex group of vitamins – B2, B5, folic acid, niacin and parabenzoic acid – beta-carotene, and the mineral zinc can all help in consolidating the process of healing. Green leafy vegetables, carrots, apricots, melons and citrus fruits are all good sources of these nutrients, and juices made with them can help.

Juices

Each recipe makes approx. one 8 fl oz/230ml glass of juice. Adults can drink up to three glasses daily, but do vary the juice combinations for maximum benefit (for children see page 49). Drink diluted if you prefer. Juice each ingredient then blend using a spoon.

4oz/125g blackcurrants
1 apple
2oz/50g raspberries

or

6oz/175g strawberries
1 mango (I prefer organic mangoes, they seem to be riper and more juicy)

or

3 large carrots
4oz/125g parsley

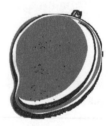

or

1 apple
6 large spinach leaves

living with added zest

Our lives seem to become busier and more pressurized every day, as we try to juggle the demands of work, family, home and leisure time. We can easily end up tired, run-down and over-stressed, and if we don't look after ourselves we can start to suffer from insomnia, digestive upsets, lack of interest in sex and a tendency to pick up minor illnesses. Fresh juices, drunk regularly, can help provide us with some of the nutrients that help us cope with stresses and strains, and enjoy life to the full.

ALERTNESS

An alert brain means you can think more quickly, concentrate better and work harder. We often turn to a cup of coffee or tea to lift that clouded feeling and bring things into clearer focus, but a fresh juice can be just as refreshing, and provide the body with valuable nutrients too. The minerals potassium, calcium, zinc and the B group of vitamins are all vital for healthy brain function.

Juices

Each recipe makes approx. one 8 fl oz/230ml glass of juice. Adults can drink up to three glasses daily, but do vary the juice combinations for maximum benefit (for children see page 49). Dilute with water if you prefer. Juice each ingredient then blend using a spoon.

1½ large carrots
7 large spinach leaves
2 stalks celery

or

2 pears
handful of watercress leaves

or

6 red cabbage leaves
¼ large cucumber
2 tomatoes

CALM VERSUS STRESS

Continuous stress and anxiety can have a very negative effect on your mental and physical health. Not only can you feel permanently fatigued and anxious, you can also experience insomnia, headaches, sore throats, poor skin, irritable bowel syndrome and sometimes more serious conditions such as stomach ulcers and heart attacks.

The immediate symptoms of stress – pounding heart, panic, tensing of muscles – are essential in the right situation. For example, if you had to escape a fire, respond to an accident, run an important race, or sit an examination, the adrenalin released into your bloodstream would provide you with the burst of energy that you needed. However, when a stressful situation occurs and there is no physical outlet for the extra energy your body supplies, stress can begin to harm your health. It puts a strain on your adrenal glands (situated behind the kidneys), which are continually producing adrenalin, and also means that you don't digest or absorb the nutrients from foods properly, because blood is diverted away from the stomach to your limbs, ready for a physical reaction. If you feel stressed frequently, perhaps every day, you will be living in a continuous state of tension and anxiety. After a while you will feel extremely drained because of an inability to relax and you may also have sleep problems.

Stress Buster

There are many things you can do to combat stress, including taking more exercise, and practising relaxation techniques such as deep breathing. But what you eat and drink can also have an effect. Nutrients which are known to have a calming effect on the nervous system are the B group of vitamins (especially B1, B6, folic acid and pantothenic acid), vitamin C, and the mineral calcium. They are found particularly in citrus fruits, green leafy vegetables, melons, apricots and avocado.

Juices

Each recipe makes approx. one 8 fl oz/230ml glass of juice. Adults can drink up to three glasses daily, but do vary the juice combinations for maximum benefit (for children see page 49). Dilute with water if you prefer. Juice each ingredient then blend using a spoon.

4oz/125g blackcurrants
1 apple

or

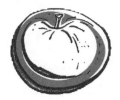

3 tangerines
6oz/175g raspberries

or

1 medium melon

or

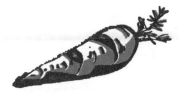

2 large carrots
1 stalk celery
4oz/125g mangetout (snow peas)

or

4oz/125g kale
¼ beetroot
4 tomatoes

Insomnia

There's nothing more infuriating than not being able to go to sleep at night, but it's one of the main side-effects of being under stress. Insomniacs often turn to sleeping pills to put them out, but fresh juices can also help: celery and lettuce juices have a reputation for helping to usher in sleep and calm the nervous system, as have juices high in the nutrients calcium and magnesium, vitamin B3 and B6.

Juices

Each recipe makes approx. one 8 fl oz/230ml glass of juice. Adults can drink up to three glasses daily, but do vary the juice combinations for maximum benefit (for children see page 49). Dilute with water if you prefer. Juice each ingredient then blend using a spoon.

4oz/125g beansprouts
4oz/125g cauliflower
2 large carrots

or

3 stalks celery
handful of watercress

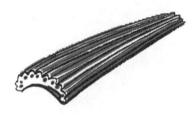

or

1 grapefruit
2 guavas

or

1 orange
6oz/175g raspberries

Fatigue

Fatigue is a debilitating result of long-term stress. You never feel rested when you wake up in the mornings, you slump in the afternoons, and feel tired again in the evenings; you seem to lack energy to do anything. Vitality-rich green juices may help to bolster up your energy levels.

Juices

Each recipe makes approx. one 8 fl oz/230ml glass of juice. Adults can drink up to three glasses daily, but do vary the juice combinations for maximum benefit (for children see page 49). Dilute with water if you prefer. Juice each ingredient then blend using a spoon.

2 large carrots
15 large spinach leaves
1 avocado, mashed

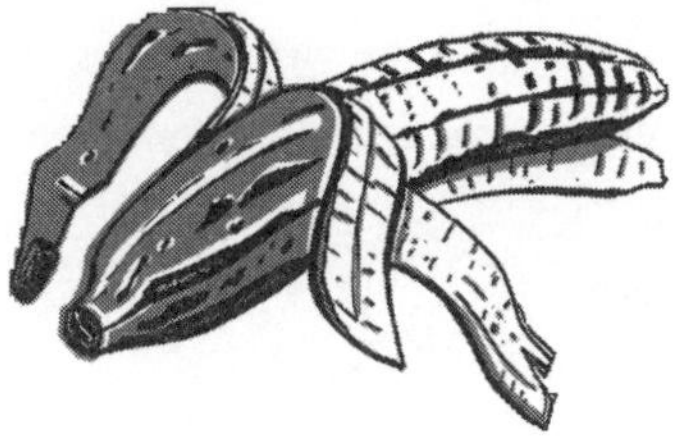

or

½ lettuce
3 stalks celery
2 tomatoes

or

2 thick slices pineapple
1 mango (I prefer organic mangoes, they seem to be riper and more juicy)
1 banana, mashed
4fl oz/115ml milk (optional)

or

1 peach
6oz/175g strawberries
1 banana, mashed
4fl oz/115ml milk

Stomach Ulcers

Stomach ulcers can be very uncomfortable and potentially life-threatening if they burst. They are often the result of stress, which can cause the stomach to secrete powerful acids even when there is no food for it to digest. Juices high in B vitamins, vitamin C and beta-carotene can be helpful, and potato and papaya juices in particular have a reputation for helping to soothe ulcers.

Juices

Each recipe makes approx. one 8 fl oz/230ml glass of juice. Adults can drink up to three glasses daily, but do vary the juice combinations for maximum benefit. Dilute with water if you prefer. Juice each ingredient then blend using a spoon.

2 large carrots
4oz/125g winter cabbage

or

2oz/50g potato
3 tomatoes

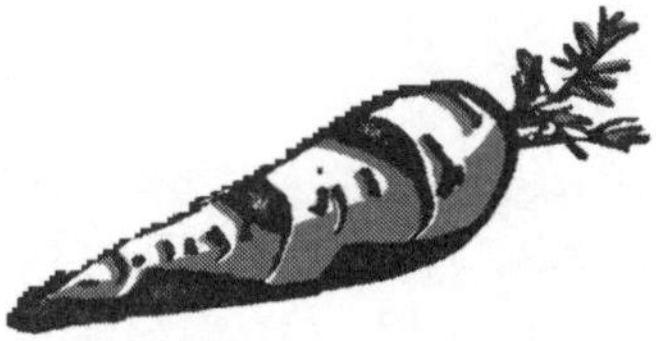

or

½ papaya
1 peach

or

¹/₂ papaya

1 apple

EXTRA ENERGY

Most fruits are sweet, as are certain vegetables like carrots and tomatoes, and make
excellent energy-giving juices. To make them even more satisfying, mix milk or plain
yoghurt with the juice recipe; you could also add some wheatgerm and honey.

Juices

Each recipe makes approx. one 8 fl oz/230ml glass of juice. Adults can drink up to three
glasses daily, but do vary the juice combinations for maximum benefit (for children see
page 49). Dilute with water if you prefer. Juice each ingredient then blend using a spoon.

1 mango (I prefer organic mangoes, they seem to be riper and more juicy)

¹/₂ medium pineapple

1 banana, mashed

¹/₄ pint milk/small pot plain yoghurt

1 tsp desiccated coconut

¹/₂ tsp honey

or

¹/₂ punnet strawberries

10 raspberries

3 apricots

4fl oz/115ml milk/yoghurt

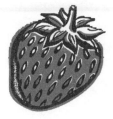

or

1 parsnip

6 white cabbage leaves

2 carrots

FRAZZLED NERVES

Do you ever find yourself in the evening with nerves frayed and temper volatile? You need to calm down, and forget about the trials of the day. Frazzled nerves can also be helped back to normality by nourishment high in the vitamin B1 (thiamine), B12 (cobalamin) and vitamin C. As vitamin B12 is not available from vegetable sources you must obtain it elsewhere (eggs, milk, cheese, beef, pork, offal).

Juices

Each recipe makes approx. one 8 fl oz/230ml glass of juice. Adults can drink up to three glasses daily, but do vary the juice combinations for maximum benefit (for children see page 49). Dilute with water if you prefer. Juice each ingredient then blend using a spoon.

½ medium watermelon

or

6 kale leaves
2 tomatoes
1 stalk celery

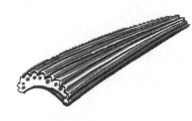

or

1 apple
1 carrot
6 Brussels sprouts

HANGOVER CURE

Hangovers are caused by two things: the toxicity of excess alcohol and dehydration. The easiest way of banishing a hangover is to flush out the alcohol from your system by drinking plenty of liquids, and to raise your energy levels by having some quick nourishment. A fresh juice combination is ideal for doing this, and can replace the vitamins B1 (thiamine) and C which are depleted by alcohol.

Juices

Each recipe makes approx. one 8 fl oz/230ml glass of juice. Adults can drink up to three glasses daily, but do vary the juice combinations for maximum benefit (for children see page 49). Dilute with water if you prefer. Juice each ingredient then blend using a spoon.

½ large pineapple
1 mango (I prefer organic mangoes, they seem to be riper and more juicy)

or

4 tangerines
1 guava

or

2 large carrots
6 kale leaves
¼ cucumber

MULTI-MINERAL BOOST

We don't need minerals in such high quantities as vitamins, but they are just as important. Some minerals are only needed in tiny trace amounts – but without them, unhealthy symptoms of deficiency soon become visible. Iron, calcium, magnesium, phosphorus, manganese, potassium, sodium and zinc are some of the minerals that we need throughout life. Vegetable juices are particularly rich in minerals and provide an excellent mineral pick-me-up.

Juices

Each recipe makes approx. one 8 fl oz/230ml glass of juice. Adults can drink up to three glasses daily, but do vary the juice combinations for maximum benefit (for children see page 49). Dilute with water if you prefer. Juice each ingredient then blend using a spoon.

1 red (bell) pepper
6 lettuce leaves
1 large carrot

or

3 tomatoes
handful of parsley
$\frac{1}{4}$ medium turnip

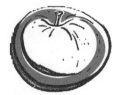

or

1 apple
$\frac{1}{4}$ beetroot
1 medium parsnip

MULTI-VITAMIN BOOST

Both children and adults need a constant supply of vitamins to stay in peak health. Juices can supply many of the nutrients we need, and in a totally natural and tasty way – more satisfying than swallowing a handful of pills. Here are some power-packed combinations for when you need that little extra vitamin boost.

Juices

Each recipe makes approx. one 8 fl oz/230ml glass of juice. Adults can drink up to three glasses daily, but do vary the juice combinations for maximum benefit (for children see page 49). Dilute with water if you prefer. Juice each ingredient then blend using a spoon.

2 large carrots
6 large spinach leaves
$\frac{1}{4}$ beetroot

or

small bunch of grapes
1 nectarine

or

2 kiwi fruits
1 pear
2 apricots

QUICK CLEANSE

Fruit and vegetable juices are ideal for detoxifying the system as they have a natural
cleansing and alkalizing effect. If taken in place of a meal they give the digestive system
a much-needed break, while still providing nutrients and energy from their natural
sugars. For more advice on detoxing with fresh juices turn to Chapter 7.

Juices

Each recipe makes approx. one 8 fl oz/230ml glass of juice. Adults can drink up to three
glasses daily, but do vary the juice combinations for maximum benefit. Dilute with water
if you prefer. Juice each ingredient then blend using a spoon.

1 apple
2 large carrots
handful of parsley

or

½ punnet strawberries
1 peach

or

1 grapefruit

1 orange

1 lemon

or

handful of wheatgrass

2 apples

1 large carrot

SEX LIFE AND APHRODISIACS

Aphrodisiacs might or might not be all in the mind — but then, nothing ventured, nothing gained. If your sex life needs a boost, perhaps you could do with some more energy, and more of the nutrients that are involved in developing and keeping healthy the reproductive organs. Juices rich in the B complex group of vitamins, vitamin E, zinc and iodine might provide you with more zest for sex. Green leafy vegetables are a good source of these nutrients. Ginseng is credited with the power to boost libido, but if ginseng root is difficult to obtain, you could use grated ginger root as an alternative — it will certainly add some spice.

Juices

Each recipe makes approx. one 8 fl oz/230ml glass of juice. Adults can drink up to three glasses daily, but do vary the juice combinations for maximum benefit. Dilute with water if you prefer. Juice each ingredient then blend using a spoon.

6oz/175g raspberries

1 nectarine

or

3 guava
4oz/125g blackberries
1 apple

or

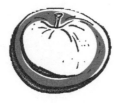

8 broccoli florets
½ red (bell) pepper
3 tomatoes

or

3 large carrots
handful of watercress

or

2 large carrots
6 lettuce leaves
1 apple
grated ginseng or ginger

RIPE OLD AGE

The elderly often require extra minerals, such as calcium, magnesium, selenium and iron, and antioxidant nutrients are also useful – vitamins C, E and beta-carotene. All vegetable and fruit juices can be a beneficial tonic.

Juices

Each recipe makes approx. one 8 fl oz/230ml glass of juice. Adults can drink up to three glasses daily, but do vary the juice combinations for maximum benefit. Dilute with water if you prefer. Juice each ingredient then blend using a spoon.

½ turnip
1 apple
6 large spinach leaves

or

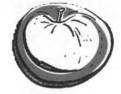

1 guava
2 peaches

or

2 large carrots
8 small broccoli florets
1 avocado, mashed

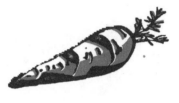

detox and revitalize

Detoxifying may be a trendy 'buzz' word, but it isn't a new concept. People have been cleansing their bodies since biblical times, often for religious reasons and to help concentrate the mind. During the twentieth century detoxification programmes have become an established treatment in addiction centres, to assist in weaning people off alcohol and drugs. Put in this context, it all sounds rather serious, but in fact detoxing is a simple and natural process that you can do in the comfort of your own home. Detoxing with fresh fruit and vegetable juices rests and rejuvenates the parts you don't normally reach – or even think about!

INTERNAL CLEANSING

Just think how much time you spend cleaning and looking after your external body. Skin is thoroughly washed, scrubbed and moisturized, hair is shampooed and conditioned, teeth are brushed and flossed day and night, tired eyes might get an eye mash on them to soothe and add sparkle.

As a clean appearance is so vitally important to most of us, shouldn't it follow that we spend time ensuring that our internal bodies are also cleansed and rested on a regular basis? After all, it is the condition of our internal organs and bloodstream that dictates whether long life and good health will be ours. Good inner health also has the added advantage of reflecting itself externally in our skin, hair, nails and eyes. It's well worth cultivating.

WHY WE NEED TO DETOX

The average modern lifestyle has its advantages, but it also has its down side too. Pollution (in the air, water and food that we eat), a poor diet, too much alcohol, smoking and stress can all contribute to a build-up of toxins in our bodies and a sluggish metabolism. Fatigue, blemishes, lacklustre hair, dull skin and eyes can all be signs that we need to eliminate toxins, rest and refresh our hard-working bodies.

A regular juice detox plan can help cleanse the blood and tissues of toxins, while providing essential nutrients for distribution around the body. Juices are particularly effective in cleansing the digestive system and the main organs of elimination: the liver, kidneys, digestive system and colon. Other methods such as body brushing, hot and cold showers, saunas and salt rubs encourage elimination via the skin (the body's biggest organ of elimination) and the lymphatic system – a network of tiny vessels which transport waste and bacteria away from cells to be neutralized or disposed of.

In addition to their cleansing powers, fresh juices provide an excellent source of vitamins, minerals and amino acids, which can replenish and strengthen existing stocks of nutrients. Juices are also easy to digest and therefore restful on the stomach and intestines, for they contain plant enzymes which aid in their breakdown.

Another important detoxifying role played by juices is their strong alkalizing effect. Like all living things, we have a pH balance between acid and alkaline. We should be more alkaline than acid, but over-acidity occurs in many of us because we eat too much protein, and sweet, fatty and processed foods. This has been linked to a weakening of the immune system, fatigue, and the overgrowth of the parasitic yeast candida albicans. Juices help to re-establish a correct pH ratio.

WHAT A DETOX PLAN INVOLVES

There are two detox plans described in this chapter – the One Day Juice Plan takes just 24 hours and is a fast (ie no food, only liquids allowed). The One Week Vitality Plan covers seven days and includes plain, natural foods as well as juices. The section entitled 'Extra Ways to Pamper Yourself' includes a number of treatments you can enjoy to enhance the detoxification process, such as body-brushing, Turkish baths and massage (see pages 119–123).

It is a good idea to start your detox plan at the weekend or on a day off. This gives you time to relax properly, sleep if you feel like it, and indulge in some of the professional therapies and home treatments suggested. If you decide to do the One Week

Vitality Plan you may have to buy and cook some foods that you wouldn't normally eat, but don't let that put you off – the results are well worth it.

Remember that the plans are guidelines, which you can adapt to suit yourself. You may stick rigidly to the plan, or you may slip up with the odd bar of chocolate or slice of pizza, but don't give up – half a detox is better than none at all. The more you get used to the concept, the easier it will become to complete a plan.

WHAT TO EXPECT

Many people find that a cleansing plan gives them more energy, and better-looking skin, hair, nails and eyes. During the One Day Juice Plan, you will undoubtedly feel hunger pangs which hopefully you can quell. You may also feel sleepy, even a little moody. If you usually drink a lot of tea and coffee, you may well develop a headache which indicates that your body is suffering withdrawal symptoms.

During the longer One Week Vitality Plan, you may experience more changes. The most common ones are unexplained mood swings, and a blow-up of blemishes or catarrh, but these indicate that your body is eliminating efficiently. As in the One Day Juice Plan, you may feel tired, or develop headaches. All these symptoms should clear up two or three days into the Plan, but if they are causing persistent discomfort then return to your normal diet.

HOW TO PREPARE

Before going on a juice detox plan, try to keep your diet as simple as possible, so that you prepare your body for the changes in store and avoid giving your digestive system a shock. Eat more fresh fruit and vegetables (raw, steamed, stir-fried), brown rice, wholewheat pasta, wholemeal bread, pulses and beans, and sprouting seeds and beans (alfalfa, mung). When breaking the plan, ease back into your normal diet gently, reintroducing foods which have been 'forbidden' only gradually.

THINGS TO AVOID

During both detox plans avoid smoking, drinking alcohol, tea, coffee, dairy products, chocolate, sugar, meat, fish, spicy foods and wheat.

FREQUENCY

If you're really keen and enjoy detoxing, you could do a One Day Juice Plan every week, but no more frequently than this. Although a juice detox is beneficial, you need to eat a well-balanced diet to keep healthy. The One Week Vitality Plan can be done once a season, or twice a year, in the summer and the winter. It should not be viewed as a permanent diet as it is too restrictive and will not provide you with a balanced diet.

EXERCISE WHILE DETOXING

Avoid intensive, competitive sports and exercise, and instead treat your body to gentle workouts such as swimming, walking and cycling. You can also practise more contemplative forms of exercise such as yoga, meditation and other relaxation techniques (see pages 119–123).

JUICE PLUS POINTS

Water is often used in detox diets, and has an important part to play in flushing out the body. But freshly made juices have several advantages over plain water. For a start, they are bursting with vitamins and minerals, and also provide energy through their simple sugars and complex carbohydrates.

Compared to pre-packed juices, fresh home-made juices contain many more nutrients. Manufacturing processes often destroy vitamins and minerals, and leave a product nutritionally depleted. Neither do fresh juices contain any extra additives such as sugar, flavourings, colourings or preservatives.

JUICE CLEANSERS

Fruit juices are stronger cleansers than vegetable juices. The strongest juices of all are made from citrus fruits, which contain high amounts of citric acid. Non-citrus fruits contain either tartaric or malic acid and have a more gentle effect. Vegetable juices are much milder in their action, and are excellent restorative drinks.

In the One Day Juice Plan, the emphasis is on fruit juices because they are stronger short-term cleansers, however, during the One Week Vitality Plan they are combined with vegetable juices for a more balanced effect. If you find that vegetable juices agree with you better, drink vegetable combinations during the One Day Juice Plan.

A WORD OF WARNING

Children, the elderly, those with diabetes and candidiasis, and those recovering from illness should not follow a detox programme without professional supervision from a naturopath/general practitioner/dietary consultant. The detox plans are **not** weight-loss diets and should not be used as such.

The best cleansing fruit juices	The best cleansing vegetable juices
Apple	Beetroot
Grape	Carrot
Grapefruit	Celery
Lemon	Cucumber
Lime	Spinach
Mango	Watercress
Melon	
Orange	
Papaya	
Peach	
Pear	
Pineapple	
Strawberry	
Watermelon	

HOW MUCH JUICE?

In both the One Day Juice Plan and the One Week Vitality Plan, you should drink up to three 8fl oz/230ml servings of juice a day, some diluted. As you become more used to the potency and effects of fresh juice, you can increase the amount to six 8fl oz/230ml servings, but to start with put the emphasis on moderation.

DETOX QUANTITY GUIDE

Here are quantities of fruit and vegetables needed to make approximately 8fl oz/230ml of undiluted juice, using a juicer

Apple Juice	10oz/275g apples or 2 medium apples
Grape Juice	10oz/275g grapes or medium bunch
Grapefruit Juice	10oz/275g grapefruit or 1½ large fruit
Mango Juice	14oz/400g mangoes or 2 mangoes
Melon Juice	12oz/350g melon or 1 medium melon
Orange Juice	10oz/275g oranges or 2 medium oranges
Papaya Juice	1lb/450g papaya or 1 large papaya
Peach Juice	12oz/350g peaches or 2 medium peaches
Pear Juice	10oz/275g pears or 2 medium pears
Pineapple Juice	14oz/400g pineapple or 1 medium one
Strawberry Juice	10oz/275g strawberries or 1 punnet
Watermelon Juice	12oz/350g melon or 1 small watermelon
Carrot Juice	14oz/400g carrots or 3 large carrots
Celery Juice	10oz/275g celery or 4 stalks
Cucumber Juice	10oz/275g cucumber or ½ a large one

Quantities of certain vegetables needed to make approximately 2fl oz/50ml of strong juice to be mixed with milder juices

Beetroot Juice	4oz/125g beetroot or ⅓ medium beet
Spinach Juice	4oz/125g spinach or 14 large leaves
Watercress Juice	4oz/125g watercress or one medium pack of leaves

Quantities of lemons and limes needed to make approximately 1fl oz/25ml juice to add to other juices

Lemon Juice   2oz/50g lemon or 1 small lemon
Lime Juice   3oz/75g lime or 1 small lime

Quantities of lemon and lime juice needed to make approximately 8fl oz/230ml of lemon or lime water

Lemon Water   squeeze of lemon in 8fl oz/230ml water
Lime Water   squeeze of lime in 8fl oz/230ml water

* Lime water is milder than lemon water and can be drunk more often as a result.

THE ONE DAY JUICE PLAN

This plan recommends the use of fruit juices only (with the exception of carrot juice, which is also an excellent liver tonifier) as they are such powerful cleansers. It is best to stick to just one type of juice throughout the day, in order to give your digestive system the least amount of work and maximum amount of rest.

You should aim to drink up to three 8fl oz/230ml servings of your chosen juice over the day, and dilute each serving with 4fl oz/115ml of water. This is because fresh juices (particularly fruit ones) are high in natural sugars, which drunk neat and without foods could make you feel a little dizzy. Drink two to three pints of other liquid during the day too. For further information on Extra Ways to Pamper Yourself during the day, turn to pages 119–123.

Choose one juice from the following list and make sure you have enough of the raw material to last you all day. Remember that in winter, soft fruits are not easily available.

Shopping List (each entry is enough for one day's juice of that particular fruit/ vegetable)

Apples	2lb/900g
Carrots	3lb/1.4kg
Grapes	2lb/900g
Grapefruit	5 large
Mangoes	6 medium
Melons	2 medium
Oranges	2lb/900g
Papaya	3 large
Peaches	2½lb/1.1kg
Pears	2lb/900g
Pineapples	3 large
Strawberries	2lb/900g

The Plan

Wake Up!

The One Day Juice Plan begins as it means to go on, with the emphasis on gentle cleansing. As soon as you wake up, drink a glass of water with a squeeze of lemon. This is an excellent way to begin the fast as it helps to cleanse the intestines.

OPTIONAL EXTRAS
Body brushing, followed by a hot shower, finished off with a burst of cold water. Afterwards give your body a good rub down with a towel, this will stimulate your circulation and lymphatic system.

Breakfast

Time for the first straight juice of the day. Drink one 8fl oz/230ml serving of juice, diluted. If you feel thirsty during the morning drink either still water, water with a squeeze of lime, or herb tea: try chamomile, lemon balm or rosehip for a soothing, cleansing effect.

OPTIONAL EXTRAS
Breathing exercises, gentle walk.

Lunch

Whenever your internal clock tells you that it's time for lunch, drink another one 8fl oz/230ml serving of your chosen juice, diluted. If you feel thirsty during the afternoon, drink water, water with a squeeze of lime, or herb teas.

OPTIONAL EXTRAS
Sauna or Turkish bath, massage.

Supper

If you have managed to keep the hunger pangs and food at bay, it's time for you to finish your fast with a flourish, and drink down the final serving of juice: drink one 8fl oz/230ml serving of juice, diluted. Drink water with a squeeze of lime, still water or herb teas if you are thirsty.

Epsom Salt Bath (if you haven't gone for a sauna or Turkish bath in the afternoon) before going to bed.

Last Thing at Night

Give your digestive system one more clean sweep by drinking a glass of water with a squeeze of lemon. Then curl up and snooze, ready to feel bright and breezy the next day.

THE ONE WEEK VITALITY PLAN

The One Week Vitality Plan combines the potency of fresh fruit and vegetable juices with plain and simple foods. This double-edged approach rests and tonifies the digestive system, while providing nourishment and strength. Regular meals are part of the plan, but the choice of food is restricted, so that maximum benefit is obtained from the cleansing programmes. Throughout the week, you can enjoy some of the Extra Ways to Pamper Yourself such as saunas, Turkish baths, massage and aromatherapy facials (see pages 119–123).

Unlike the One Day Juice Plan, this programme includes vegetable juices too, so that you gain maximum nutritional benefit from their wide range of nutrients. Below are a range of seven different juice cocktails, which are combinations of complementary juices, one variety of every day. Drink no more than one 8fl oz/230ml serving of the day's juice (diluted if you prefer), half an hour before breakfast, lunch and supper.

Refer to the shopping list below for advice on quantities of fruit and vegetables needed for juicing. If you cannot obtain one of the fruits listed in a cocktail, simply replace that cocktail with the Apple and Carrot Bomber (see page 114). If pears are out of season, use apples, grapes or pineapple instead. Make sure that you drink two to three pints of other liquids each day.

Shopping List for a Week's Juices

Apples	3lb/1.4kg
Beetroot	1½lb/675g
Carrots	4lb/1.8kg
Celery	1 head (bunch)
Grapes	1lb/450g
Grapefruit	3 large
Mangoes	2 large
Oranges	1lb/450g
Pineapples	2 large
Spinach	1lb/450g

JUICES FOR THE WEEK

Day 1

Apple and Carrot Bomber

4fl oz/115ml apple juice

4fl oz/115ml carrot juice

DAY 2

Grapefruit Guzzle

5fl oz/145ml grapefruit juice

3fl oz/80ml orange juice

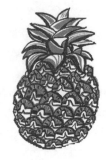

DAY 3

Big on Beetroot

2fl oz/50ml beetroot juice

6fl oz/170ml apple juice

DAY 4

Tropical Twist

5fl oz/145ml pineapple juice

3fl oz/80ml mango juice (I prefer organic mangoes, they seem to be riper and more juicy)

DAY 5

Super Spinach

4fl oz/115ml carrot juice

2fl oz/50ml spinach juice

2fl oz/50ml celery juice

DAY 6

Big Apple

5fl oz/145ml apple juice
3fl oz/80ml grape juice

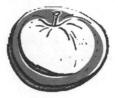

DAY 7

Blushing Beetroot

6fl oz/170ml carrot juice
2fl oz/50ml beetroot juice

FOODS DURING THE WEEK

The choice of foods in the One Week Vitality Plan is deliberately limited, although nutritious and filling so you won't go hungry. The restrictions increase the cleansing power of the diet, and give your overworked digestive system a much-needed rest. Key elements are wholegrains such as brown rice, barley and millet, which can be steamed or gently boiled and then seasoned with fresh herbs, soy sauce and lemon juice; and fresh fruit and vegetables that can be steamed, stir-fried or eaten raw.

Basic Breakfast Foods

Fresh whole fruits or fruit salad
Porridge (made with jumbo oats, water and a handful of raisins or a chopped banana
    for sweetness)

Basic Lunch Foods

Mixed salad: select from lettuce, white cabbage, red cabbage, tomato, beansprouts,
    alfalfa, chickpeas, watercress, grated carrot, fennel, radish, celery, green and red
    (bell) peppers
Steamed or stir-fried vegetables
Fresh fruit
Cooked brown rice, millet or barley, seasoned if preferred

Basic Supper Foods

Steamed, raw or stir-fried vegetables
Mixed salad (selection as above)
Fresh fruits
Cooked brown rice, millet or barley, seasoned if preferred

Anytime Snack Foods

Sea vegetables (kombu, wakame and dulse seaweeds are very nutritious)

Rice cakes

Oat cakes

Hummus

Tahini spread

Raisins

Pumpkin seeds

Sunflower seeds

Crudités (carrot, cucumber, red [bell] pepper, cauliflower)

Alternative Drinks

Herb teas

Still water

Water with a squeeze of lime added

THE PLAN

Wake Up!

Open those bleary eyes and drink down a glass of water with a squeeze of lemon.

OPTIONAL EXTRAS
Body brushing and a hot, then cold shower.

Breakfast

Drink one 8fl oz/230ml serving of juice (diluted if preferred) half an hour before you eat. Then tuck into breakfast.

OPTIONAL EXTRA
Meditation (see page 121).

Lunch

Drink one 8fl oz/230ml serving of juice (diluted if preferred), half an hour before you eat. Then eat lunch.

OPTIONAL EXTRA
Gentle exercise, e.g. a walk, swim or yoga.

Supper

Drink your final 8fl oz/230ml serving of the juice cocktail of the day, half an hour before food. Then eat supper.

Last Thing at Night

Drink a glass of water with a squeeze of lemon juice to cleanse the digestive tract.

EXTRA WAYS TO PAMPER YOURSELF

A variety of extra activities such as saunas, mud packs and massage provide welcome distractions from tempting chocolate bars and alluring pizzas. At the end of this section you will find an easy chart which you can refer to for integrating treatments into a detox plan.

Body Brushing

Body brushing stimulates the lymphatic system (the tiny network of vessels which clear waste from the cells), and also the circulation. It only takes five minutes to do, and is very effective in removing dry skin, especially on the legs. You can use a natural bristle brush or a dry wash cloth, or a dry loofah: simply apply it to the skin on your feet and make small, circular strokes, moving up your legs, always working upwards in the direction of the heart area. Once you've reached this part of the body, move to the top of the neck and brush downwards to the heart. Body brushing is most effective when followed by a warm bath or shower.

Salt Rub

This treatment will make your skin tingle as it stimulates your blood circulation. You will need a pack of coarse-grain sea-salt, a wash cloth or bath brush, and a shower. Have your warm shower as usual, then turn off the water. Throw some sea salt on to your legs and rub briskly with the cloth or brush, and gradually work up your body, throwing on more salt (always work towards the heart). Then rinse off salt with lukewarm water. Salt rubs are not suitable for those with eczema or psoriasis.

Epsom Salt Bath

Epsom salt baths are easy to enjoy at home and very relaxing, but do not use if you suffer from high blood-pressure, eczema or psoriasis. In addition, they should not be used in combination with a salt rub (see above), or your skin will become very dry. Epsom salts contain magnesium sulphate and help to draw impurities from the skin. Add ½lb–1lb (225–450g) of salts to a hot bath and soak for 15–20 minutes. When you get out of the bath, keep warm by wrapping up in thick clothes or going to bed. For several hours afterwards, your body will continue to perspire and eliminate toxins from the skin. Epsom Salts are available from chemists and some health food stores; if you can't get hold of them you could use ordinary bath salts instead.

Sauna

The dry heat of a sauna encourages the body to sweat and eliminate impurities through the skin. Some people can stay in a sauna for 20 minutes at a stretch, others heat up much more quickly. As soon as you start to feel uncomfortable or your heart begins to pound, leave the sauna room, shower off and cool down. After five to ten minutes you'll probably feel ready to go back in again, but an hour to an hour and a half altogether is usually enough time in a sauna.

Turkish Bath

Hot, humid and jungle-steamy, a Turkish bath is an experience not to be missed. A series of communal areas range in temperatures and humidity, all designed to produce sweat by the bucketful and help flush out impurities. In between relaxing in each area, you are supposed to shower off under a cold jet of water, or jump into an icy-cold plunge pool. This closes pores and improves blood circulation. Masseurs are usually available to scrub and massage your body if you wish.

Aromatherapy Massage

This form of massage combines the technique of body massage with the use of essential plant oils. Massage is most satisfying when someone else is doing it for you, but you can do self-massage too. All you need is a bottle of almond oil and an essential oil of your choice. Pour out an eggcupful of almond oil and add a couple of drops of essential oil (eg lavender, ylang ylang or rosemary). Using smooth strokes, massage it into your skin.

Meditation

For a tranquil start to your day, try a little meditation. If possible sit cross-legged on the floor, shut your eyes and breathe in deeply and slowly. Hold your breath for a few seconds, then let it out slowly. Repeat the sequence twice. Now picture a calm and beautiful scene and concentrate on it, feeling the pleasure and energy it generates. Continue for five to ten minutes, then gently rouse yourself.

Body Scrunching

Lie on the floor face up and gradually tense up all your muscles and hold for ten seconds, then release, and repeat twice. Remain lying down, but place a book under your head. Draw your feet up towards your body, so that they are just below your knees. Feel your hips and spine sinking into the floor and gently stretching and realigning. Vapours from an oil burner, coupled with the sound of relaxing music, can enhance the atmosphere.

Facial Steam

Give your face a cleansing boost with a facial steam. All you need is a heavy-based bowl, some just-boiled water, a towel and a bottle of essential oil such as lavender, ylang ylang or geranium. Fill the bowl half-full with the water and add two drops of essential oil. Then place your head over the bowl and cover it with a towel. Steam for five to ten minutes. This will open pores and make it easier to extract blackheads and dirt from your skin. If you have time afterwards, smooth on a face mask and cover your eyes with two slices of cucumber (very soothing to tired eyes). Then wash off the mask, cleanse, tone and moisturize.

Manicure

Make your hands look fit for a queen by giving them a home manicure treat. Trim and file ragged nails, then soak your hands in a bowl of warm soapy water for a couple of minutes. Pat them dry with a towel and push back cuticles with an orange stick. Massage in a rich cuticle cream and leave for a few minutes, wipe off excess cream, then for a spot of real glamour you can paint your nails a glossy colour (use a neutral base coat first to avoid staining the nails).

Hair Treatment

Your hand and scalp deserve a bit of special treatment just as much as any other part of your body. First of all, why not give yourself a relaxing massage, to get rid of those tight bands of tension. Starting at the bottom of your neck, place your fingertips against your skin and move upwards on to the head. Make kneading patterns over your neck and head – be firm, it works better. If your scalp is dry use a little almond oil to help moisturize it. Now wash and condition your hair. If you have time, use a deep action conditioner and wrap your hair up in a towel while it goes into action. Then rinse hair and blow dry.

NOTE
For more detailed information on detoxing and further detox plans see my book *The Juicing Detox Diet*, also published by Thorsons.

Choose from these suggested Extra Ways to Pamper Yourself

Suggested Treatment	The One Day Juice Plan	The One Week Vitality Plan
Body Brushing	once	every day
Salt Rub/Epsom Salt Bath (shouldn't be done on separate days; not suitable for eczema or psoriasis sufferers	once	once
Sauna	once	once
Turkish Bath	once	once
Aromatherapy Massage	once	once
Meditation	once	every day
Body Scrunching	once	every day
Facial Steam	once	once
Manicure	once	once
Hair Treatment	once	once
Gentle Exercise	once	every day

juice it up!

the fresh juice bar

While ultra-fresh juices enhance wellbeing, they can also be made into a delicious range of drinks that taste as good as they look. Pick and choose from the 'Fresh Juice Bar' and discover how easy it is to make smoothies – some so filling they make great breakfast or lunch replacements; delicious straight juice combos; cocktails with a kick; and juices just for kids. Try them out, adjust to taste, and you'll soon be coming up with your own favourite blends.

All fresh juice blends and smoothies are best drunk straightaway, however if you do want to take one on a day out or into work, add a squeeze of lemon juice to the mix – this will stop the fruit/vegetables from oxidising and turning brown. Transport in a Thermos flask to keep chilled and shake gently before pouring.

If you prefer smoothies and juice blends chilled – I do – keep the ingredients in the fridge and/or whizz up some icecubes together with your chosen drink.

CUSTOMISING JUICE BLENDS

It's fun and easy to add extra ingredients to smoothies and juices. These extras can add piquancy, flavour, nutrients and of course extra calories – if you want them.

Citrus Zest

When using citrus fruits, why not grate a little of the zest from the outer skin and sprinkle into your juice; lime and lemon zest are particularly flavoursome (but make sure to give the fruit a good scrub beforehand).

Spices and Herbs

Spices can add wonderful flavour to many fruit and vegetable juices, and you can use them fresh or dried. Fresh spices and herbs such as ginger, nutmeg, coriander (cilantro), basil, oregano, thyme, mint, parsley, rosemary, chilli pepper and dill can be put through the juicer along with other produce, or you can grate or chop them very finely and add to the glass after juicing.

If fresh spices and herbs aren't available you might like to sprinkle some dried spices into your juice. For fruit juices pick from cinnamon, nutmeg, ginger and allspice. For vegetable juices choose from ginger, coriander, fennel, fenugreek, cumin, cardamom, saffron and turmeric, basil, oregano, mint, thyme, parsley, rosemary and dill; you can even add a spot of chilli powder, chilli sauce or Tabasco sauce for red hot flavour. Worcester sauce, salt and freshly ground black pepper can also make a really tasty difference.

Milk and Ice-Cream

Make long, refreshing fruity milkshakes by adding half a pint of milk (cow's, sheep, soya) to 5fl oz/145ml of your favourite fruit juice. Whip up in a blender, if possible, to produce that tempting frothy look. For real indulgence, turn your juice milkshake into a luxurious float by adding a couple of scoops of your favourite ice-cream.

Yoghurt

Plain yoghurt makes an excellent accompaniment to fruit juices; Greek-style gives a lovely creamy texture, and live yoghurt contains beneficial bacteria which colonize the gut. See page 187 for a recipe on how to make your own yoghurt with added fruit pulp.

Honey

Although fruit juices are naturally sweet, you can also add half a teaspoonful of honey or even blend in a little honey comb if you prefer. Providing extra natural sugar might give you more of an instant pep up.

Blended Fruit

Mashed banana blended with fruit juice adds great flavour and makes a juice into an energy-rich drink. You can also blend soft summer fruits like raspberries, strawberries, apricots, peaches, blackberries, loganberries, cranberries, kiwi fruit, pineapple, blackcurrants and redcurrants. If you have a food processor, just pour in the juice and add the whole fruit, blend and serve – it tastes delicious.

For vegetable juices, mashed avocado is the banana equivalent, adding flavour and supplying extra energy when blended in with a juice. Blending in finely chopped spring onion or cherry tomatoes gives extra zing; to bolster vitamin and mineral content add a handful of lettuce, watercress or baby spinach leaves to the juicer, as you juice your chosen vegetables.

Coconut and Wheatgerm

The addition of fresh desiccated coconut, or cream or milk, gives fruit juices a delicious tropical taste. Add a dessertspoonful to any juice you choose. Wheatgerm provides extra fibre and vitamin E; just as you might sprinkle it over your cereal, add a teaspoon to a glass of juice.

Sprouts

Sprouts from dried seeds and pulses such as alfalfa, fenugreek, radish, mung beans, aduki beans, chick peas and lentils make a highly nutritious addition to vegetable juice blends. Sprouts are rich in enzymes and chlorophyll which aid digestion. You can either put them through the juicer at the same time as your chosen vegetables or whizz them up in the blender with the ready-juiced vegetables (this way provides the greatest health benefit). You can buy mung bean sprouts ready-grown from most supermarkets (look for Chinese-style bean sprouts). For a wider range of ready-grown sprouts visit your local whole food/health food store.

Growing your own Sprouts

Of course it's much cheaper and really rather satisfying to grow your own! All you need to get going is a pack of seeds or beans (purchase from a whole food store) and a sprouting jar (either a wide-mouthed jam jar or a special sprouting jar – available very reasonably from some whole food stores). Note that each quantity of seeds/beans you grow will yield approximately eight times that amount of sprouts, so don't overfill your jar.

1 First choose your sprout, then rinse a handful of the dried seeds/pulses under the tap.
2 Once thoroughly rinsed, place them in the sprouting jar and cover them with a couple of inches of water. To protect the sprouts from dust, but allow them to breathe, place a double layer of muslin (alternatively drape with a tea towel), secured with a rubber band, over the top of the jar and leave to soak overnight somewhere dark, such as a kitchen cupboard, to encourage germination.
3 The following morning drain off the water and rinse the sprouts again. Shake off excess water, and replace in the jar (the sprouts should be damp but not water-logged). Return the jar to its dark resting place.
4 Repeat the rinsing process morning and evening for another three to five days (depending on the type of seed/pulse) and return jar to dark place afterwards.
5 As the sprouts become ready to eat – you'll know because their curly tendrils will have zoomed up a centimetre or two from the seed/pulse husk – place them on a windowsill for a few hours of sunshine.
6 Before adding to juice, rinse sprouts again; if you prefer to remove the husks, place the sprouts in a full bowl of water, stir, and the husks should float to the top.

Sprouting Ready Reckoner*

* Alfalfa – ready in 6 days
* Fenugreek – ready in 4 days
* Radish – ready in 5 days
* Mung beans – ready in 5 days
* Aduki beans – ready in 5 days

* Chickpeas – ready in 4 days

* Lentils – ready in 5 days

(* Sprouts may be ready a day or so earlier, depending on vigour of growth.)

Water

If you prefer your juices diluted you can add still or sparkling water, or even soda water and have a fresh juice spritzer! Children should always drink juices half diluted with water. For a slush effect, crunch up some ice cubes (wrap in a tea-towel and roll with a rolling pin), and add to your juice.

All Dressed Up!

If you want to make your juices look special, invest in some cocktail sticks or swizzle sticks, cocktail umbrellas, bendy straws and colourful fresh fruit like cherries, kiwi fruit, pineapple, raspberries and strawberries to slice up and decorate the glass. Find a chunky glass, put sliced fruit on cocktail/swizzle sticks, add a paper umbrella and you've got a colourful and exotic juice drink. For that extra bit of professionalism, why not sugar-frost the glasses. Simply rub the rim of the glass with a piece of fruit (eg mango, grape), then lightly roll it in a saucer of white sugar.

SUPER SMOOTHIES

Use banana, ice cream, milk, freshly squeezed orange juice and unjuiced fruit flesh to create a heavenly range of smoothies.

Berry Smoothie

MAKES APPROX. ONE 8FL OZ/230ML SERVING

1 apple
5 large strawberries
10 raspberries
10 blackberries

Juice the apple, then pour into a blender, add the strawberries, raspberries and blackberries and whip up. Pour into a glass.

Pineapple and Pear Perfection

MAKES APPROX. ONE 8FL OZ/230ML SERVING

1 pear
1 apple
1 thick slice of pineapple, skinned and chopped

Juice the pear and apple and pour into a blender, add the chopped up pineapple (skin removed) and whip up. Serve.

Papaya Smoothie

MAKES APPROX. ONE 8FL OZ/230ML SERVING

1½ apples
½ lime
piece of root ginger (approx. ½ inch/1 cm square)
½ papaya (remove black seeds)

Juice the apples, lime and ginger together, pour into a blender and add the papaya flesh. Blend, then serve.

Pink Mango

MAKES APPROX. ONE 8FL OZ/230ML SERVING

1 pink grapefruit

1 apple

½ mango (I prefer organic mangoes, they seem to be riper and more juicy)

Juice the grapefruit and apple, pour into a blender. Add the mango flesh. Blend, then serve.

Passion Juice

MAKES APPROX. ONE 8FL OZ/230ML SERVING

3 ruby oranges

½ lime

1 passion fruit

Juice the oranges and the lime, pour into a blender. Add the passion fruit flesh. Blend, then serve.

Banana and Pear Shake

MAKES APPROX. ONE 8FL OZ/230ML SERVING

2 small pears

1 banana, mashed

30fl oz/80ml milk

Juice the pears, pour into a blender. Add the banana and milk. Blend, then serve.

Carrot Smoothie

MAKES APPROX. ONE 8FL OZ/230ML SERVING
2 large carrots
1 avocado, mashed
sprig of coriander (cilantro), chopped

Juice the carrots and pour into a blender. Add the avocado and coriander. Blend and serve.

Green Wonder

MAKES APPROX. ONE 8FL OZ/230ML SERVING
1 stalk celery
6 kale leaves
2 tomatoes
½ avocado, mashed
sprig of fresh oregano, chopped

Juice the celery, kale and tomatoes. Pour into a blender. Add the avocado and oregano. Blend and serve.

Apricot Smoothie

MAKES APPROX. ONE 8FL OZ/230ML SERVING
Juice and blend:
3 apricots
2fl oz/50ml yoghurt
4fl oz/115ml milk

Mango Milkshake

MAKES APPROX. ONE 8FL OZ/230ML SERVING

Juice and blend:

1 mango (I prefer organic mangoes, they seem to be riper and more juicy)

1 nectarine

5fl oz/145ml milk

Strawberry Ice

MAKES APPROX. ONE 8FL OZ/230ML SERVING

8 strawberries

1 scoop frozen Greek yoghurt

3fl oz/80ml milk

Thoroughly blend all the ingredients, then serve. Add crushed ice to taste.

Banana Passion

MAKES APPROX. ONE 8FL OZ/230ML SERVING

1 passion fruit

1 large orange, freshly squeezed

1 banana, mashed

1 level tsp honey (optional)

Scoop out the seeds from the passion fruit and place in a blender with the mashed banana and freshly squeezed orange juice. Blend thoroughly. If the Smoothie is a little too tart, add honey to taste, then serve.

Al's Super Zinger

1 crunchy apple
1 mango (I prefer organic mangoes, they seem to be riper and more juicy)
1 passion fruit
juice of ½ lime, squeezed
2 icecubes

Juice the apple and, along with the other ingredients, place in a blender. Blend thoroughly, then serve.

Soya Shake

MAKES APPROX. ONE 8FL OZ/230ML SERVING
1 mango (I prefer organic mangoes, which seem to be riper and more juicy)
handful of blueberries
4fl oz/115ml soya milk, chilled
1 scoop soya milk vanilla icecream (optional)

Place all the ingredients in a blender. For an extra creamy taste, add a scoop of icecream. Blend thoroughly, then serve.

Shades of Summer

MAKES APPROX. ONE 8FL OZ/230ML SERVING
2 oranges, freshly squeezed
handful of blackberries
handful of raspberries
2 icecubes

Place the freshly squeezed orange juice, together with the blackberries and raspberries into a blender. Add a couple of icecubes. Blend thoroughly, then serve.

Peachy Sweet

MAKES APPROX. ONE 8FL OZ/230ML SERVING
1 ripe peach

1 ripe nectarine

1 orange

1 scoop frozen Greek yoghurt

Juice the peach, nectarine and orange. Place in a blender with the frozen yoghurt, blend thoroughly, then serve.

BIG SMOOTHIES

These smoothies are power-packed to make an easy-to-digest vitality snack – or see you through a light lunch.

Caribbean Milk Shake

MAKES APPROX. ONE 8FL OZ/230ML SERVING
½ large pineapple

milk of 1 coconut

fresh, grated coconut

1 banana, mashed

grated nutmeg

3fl oz/80ml milk

Juice the pineapple (reserving one chunk for decoration) and pour into a blender, add the coconut milk, grated coconut, mashed banana and milk. Blend. Pour into a glass and sprinkle with nutmeg. For fun decorate with a swizzle stick and the chunk of pineapple, and a paper umbrella.

Pink Sunset Float

MAKES APPROX. ONE 8FL OZ/230ML SERVING
½ papaya
½ mango (I prefer organic mangoes, they seem to be riper and more juicy)
1 banana, mashed
1 tbsp live yoghurt
3fl oz/8oz milk or a scoop of vanilla ice-cream

Juice the papaya and pour into a blender. Add the mango flesh, banana, yoghurt and milk (or ice-cream). Blend and serve.

Mango and Peach Lassi

MAKES APPROX. ONE 8FL OZ/230ML SERVING
1 peach
½ mango (I prefer organic mangoes, they seem to be riper and more juicy)
3fl oz/80ml Greek yoghurt
1 tsp honey
1 tsp wheatgerm
3fl oz/80ml milk

Juice the peach, pour into a blender. Add the mango flesh, Greek yoghurt, honey, wheatgerm and milk. Blend, then serve.

Cucumber and Avocado Lassi

MAKES APPROX. ONE 8FL OZ/230ML SERVING
½ small cucumber
fresh mint, chopped
½ avocado, mashed
2fl oz/50ml Greek yoghurt

Decoration:
2 thin slices of cucumber
sprig of fresh mint

Juice the cucumber and pour into a blender. Add the fresh mint, avocado and Greek yoghurt. Blend and serve, decorate with a mint sprig and two slices of cucumber.

Banana Bounty

MAKES APPROX. ONE 8FL OZ/230ML SERVING
Juice and blend:
1 mango (I prefer organic mangoes, they seem to be riper and more juicy)
2 thick slices pineapple
1 banana, mashed
5fl oz/145ml milk

Orange, Banana and Raspberry Smoothie

MAKES APPROX. ONE 8FL OZ/230ML SERVING
Juice and blend:
1 large orange
1 banana, mashed
8 raspberries
1 tsp wheatgerm

Blueberry Blast

MAKES APPROX. ONE 8FL OZ/230ML SERVING
handful of blueberries

1 banana, mashed

2 scoops vanilla icecream

4fl oz/115ml milk

Place all the ingredients in a blender. Blend thoroughly, then serve.

In the Pink

MAKES APPROX. ONE 8FL OZ/230ML SERVING
1 papaya, deseeded

1 banana, mashed

handful of strawberries

3fl oz/80ml chilled milk (or soya milk, if you prefer)

Juice the papaya and, together with the other ingredients, place in a blender. Blend thoroughly, then serve.

Super 'A'

MAKES APPROX. ONE 8FL OZ/230ML SERVING
large handful of baby spinach leaves

2 large carrots

1 apple

1 papaya

2 ice cubes

Juice the carrots and spinach leaves together, then the apple. Place in a blender with the papaya and ice cubes and blend thoroughly, then serve.

Delicious Fig

MAKES APPROX. ONE 8FL OZ/230ML SERVING

2 oranges

1 banana, mashed

flesh of 3 plump figs

Juice the oranges and, together with the banana and fig flesh, place in a blender. Blend thoroughly, then serve.

JUST JUICES

Juice on juice – how much more tempting can a blend get? And so good for you too...

MAKE A MEAL OF IT

Juices are an excellent accompaniment to breakfast, lunch and supper. If you're new to juicing, don't drink more than three 8fl oz/230ml glasses a day – or your tummy won't know what's hit it! As you become more accustomed to the concentrated power of juices you can increase this to between four and six glasses a day. Always remember that it is much more beneficial to vary your juice recipes (even over one day) so that you drink both fruit and vegetable juices and balance the goodness from both types. (For more details about juices for children see page 49). Here are some easy recipes to tickle your tastebuds.

Breakfast Juices

These can be drunk on their own or with breakfast foods, but do remember that (wo)man cannot survive on juices alone! If you have time, drink your juice half an hour before you eat breakfast, to give it time to be well absorbed.

Grape Ripple

MAKES APPROX. ONE 8FL OZ/230ML SERVING
1½ apples
20 white grapes
10 red grapes

Juice the apples and white grapes and pour into a glass. Then juice the red grapes and pour into the glass to achieve a ripple effect.

King Kiwi

MAKES APPROX. ONE 8FL OZ/230ML SERVING
2 small pears
1 kiwi fruit
½ mango (I prefer organic mangoes, they seem to be riper and more juicy)
sprig of mint, chopped

Juice the pears, kiwi fruit and mango, pour into a blender and add the chopped mint. Blend, then serve.

Golden Carrot

MAKES APPROX. ONE 8FL OZ/230ML SERVING
1 small orange
1 small apple
2 large carrots
½ lime
piece of root ginger (approx. ½ inch/1cm square)

Juice the orange, apple, carrots, lime and ginger, pour into a blender. Blend and serve.

Carrot Zinger

MAKES APPROX. ONE 8FL OZ/230ML SERVING

1 tomato

2 sticks celery

2 large carrots

$\frac{1}{2}$ lemon

sprig of parsley

Juice the tomato, celery, carrots and lemon. Pour into glass and add a sprig of fresh parsley.

Beetroot Slammer

MAKES APPROX. ONE 8FL OZ/230ML SERVING

$\frac{1}{2}$ apple

2 large carrots

$\frac{1}{4}$ raw beetroot

piece of root ginger (approx. $\frac{1}{2}$ inch/1cm square)

$\frac{1}{2}$ lime

sprig of coriander (cilantro)

Juice the apple, carrots, beetroot, ginger and lime. Blend and serve decorated with a sprig of coriander.

Thai Spice

MAKES APPROX. ONE 8FL OZ/230ML SERVING

$\frac{1}{4}$ large cucumber

2 large carrots

$\frac{1}{2}$ lime

1 red chilli

sprig of coriander (cilantro)

Juice the cucumber, carrots, lime and chilli. Blend and serve in a glass decorated with the sprig of coriander (cilantro).

Watercress Whizz

MAKES APPROX. ONE 8FL OZ/230ML SERVING
2 tomatoes
¼ large cucumber
handful of watercress
sprig of basil, chopped

Juice the tomatoes, cucumber and watercress. Blend and pour into a glass, decorate with chopped basil.

Pepper Up!

MAKES APPROX. ONE 8FL OZ/230ML SERVING
1 carrot
1 red (bell) pepper
4oz/125g chunk of red cabbage
sprig of fresh thyme, chopped

Juice the carrot, red pepper and red cabbage. Blend and add the chopped thyme, then serve.

St Clement's

MAKES APPROX. ONE 8FL OZ/230ML SERVING
Juice and blend:
1 orange
1 grapefruit
½ lemon

Kiwi Cooler

MAKES APPROX. ONE 8FL OZ/230ML SERVING
Juice and blend:

2 kiwi fruit

1½ large apples

Pear Drop

MAKES APPROX. ONE 8FL OZ/230ML SERVING
Juice and blend:

2 small pears

2 thick slices of pineapple

Super Carrot

MAKES APPROX. ONE 8FL OZ/230ML SERVING
Juice and blend:

3 large carrots

handful of watercress

sprig of coriander (cilantro)

Tomato Bliss

MAKES APPROX. ONE 8FL OZ/230ML SERVING
Juice and blend:

3 tomatoes

2 stalks of celery

sprig of coriander (cilantro)

Lunchtime Juices

There's nothing like a flask of fresh juice to look forward to at the midday break. Try these lunchtime lifters.

Simply Strawberry

MAKES APPROX. ONE 8FL OZ/230ML SERVING
Juice and blend:
½ punnet strawberries
1 peach

Peak Papaya

MAKES APPROX. ONE 8FL OZ/230ML SERVING
Juice and blend:
½ papaya
2 small pears

Cucumber Combo

MAKES APPROX. ONE 8FL OZ/230ML SERVING
Juice and blend:
¼ large cucumber
4 broccoli florets
2 tomatoes

Carrot and Coriander

MAKES APPROX. ONE 8FL OZ/230ML SERVING
Juice and blend:
3 large carrots
several sprigs of coriander (cilantro)

Sergeant Pepper

MAKES APPROX. ONE 8FL OZ/230ML SERVING
Juice and blend:
½ red (bell) pepper
½ green (bell) pepper
2 large carrots

Supper Juices

Put your feet up, glass of juice in hand, and gently unwind before supper. Try these tempting recipes.

Melon Refresher

MAKES APPROX. ONE 8FL OZ/230ML SERVING
Juice and blend:
1 small melon
sprinkle of cinnamon

Gentle Grapefruit

MAKES APPROX. ONE 8FL OZ/230ML SERVING
Juice and blend:
1½ grapefruit
1 lime

Cool Carrot

MAKES APPROX. ONE 8FL OZ/230ML SERVING
Juice and blend:

2 large carrots

¼ head celeriac

4oz/125g chunk red cabbage

Beetnik

MAKES APPROX. ONE 8FL OZ/230ML SERVING
Juice and blend:

2 large carrots

⅓ medium beetroot

2 sprigs of fresh basil

Tomato Toner

MAKES APPROX. ONE 8FL OZ/230ML SERVING
Juice and blend:

3 tomatoes

¼ large cucumber

6 spinach leaves

Christmas Cranberry

MAKES APPROX. ONE 8FL OZ/230ML SERVING
4 tangerines

handful of cranberries

Juice both ingredients. Place both in a blender and blend thoroughly, then serve.

Cranberry Twist

MAKES APPROX. ONE 8FL OZ/230ML SERVING
3 large carrots
handful of cranberries
squeeze of lime

Juice the carrots together with the cranberries and squeeze of lime juice. Blend thoroughly, then serve.

JUICES JUST FOR KIDS

Juices can be just as good for children as they can for adults, but in lesser quantities. Because fresh juices are so concentrated they also need to be diluted by at least half for children, or they may overpower young digestive systems. Stick to these guidelines:

- Children from 3 to 12 years of age, no more than 5fl oz/145ml fresh juice a day, diluted.
- Teenagers can start drinking undiluted juice, but stick to one to two 8fl oz/230ml servings a day.
- Avoid giving very strong juices such as spinach, watercress, parsley and beetroot to children, or if you do just include a couple of leaves or one or two thin slices and mix with a milder juice such as carrot or apple.

Start off by giving your child perhaps three or four servings of diluted juice a week, slowly building up to one or two servings a day if they like them (remember, no more than 5fl oz/145ml total fresh juice a day). Try single juices first, diluted by at least half, then as they become more accustomed to the taste you can combine juices (still diluting them). For the greatest benefit, make sure children drink a variety of juices each week.

A juice with added mashed banana or avocado not only quenches thirst, but can act as a healthy between-meals snack too.

Young Children

The following juices are tempting to small tastebuds; the quantity given in each case is that needed to make 5fl oz/145ml fresh juice, but always dilute by at least half with still water or milk.

Apple	1 large
Apricot	4
Carrot	2 large
Celery	2 stalks
Cucumber	1/3 large cucumber
Grapefruit	1 large
Mango	1 large
Orange	1 large
Pear	2 small
Pineapple	1/2 medium
Raspberry	3/4 punnet
Strawberry	3/4 punnet
Tangerine	4
Tomato	3 tomatoes
Watermelon	1/2 medium

Older Children

Try these juice combinations for older children and teenagers. As you become more experienced in making them you can devise your own juice recipes. Remember that apple and carrot are the only juices that can be satisfactorily mixed with either fruit or vegetable juices; and that melon (including watermelon) should be drunk on its own, as it goes through the digestive system much faster than other juices.

Bright Eyes

MAKES APPROX. 10FL OZ/300ML
Juice and blend:
1 apple
1 carrot
5fl oz/145ml still water

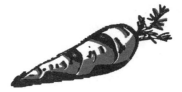

Sweet Pear

MAKES APPROX. 10FL OZ/300ML
Juice and blend:
1 pear
handful of strawberries
5fl oz/145ml still water

Raspberry Sparkle

MAKES APPROX. 10FL OZ/300ML
Juice and blend:
handful of raspberries
1 large orange
5fl oz/145ml still water

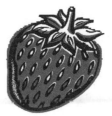

Watermelon Wonder

MAKES APPROX. 10FL OZ/300ML
Juice and blend:
large slice of watermelon
5fl oz/145ml still water

Tangerine Tickler

MAKES APPROX. 10FL OZ/300ML

Juice and blend:

3 tangerines

1 guava

5fl oz/145ml still water

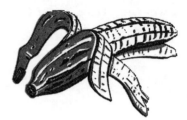

Pineapple and Banana Smoothie

MAKES APPROX. 10FL OZ/300ML

Juice and blend:

2 thick slices of pineapple

1 banana, mashed

5fl oz/145ml milk

Blackberry Hollow

MAKES APPROX. 10FL OZ/300ML

Juice and blend:

3oz/75g blackberries

3oz/75g strawberries

5fl oz/145ml still water

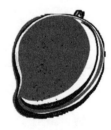

Mango Tango Smoothie

MAKES APPROX. 10FL OZ/300ML

Juice and blend:

1 mango (I prefer organic mangoes, they seem to be riper and more juicy)

1 banana, mashed

5fl oz/145ml milk

Apple Whizz

MAKES APPROX. 10FL OZ/300ML

Juice and blend:

3oz/75g raspberries

1 apple

5fl oz/145ml still water

Grapefruit Sun Splash

MAKES APPROX. 10FL OZ/300ML

Juice and blend:

1 grapefruit

1 orange

6 cherries

5fl oz/145ml still water

Tomato Topper

MAKES APPROX. 10FL OZ/300ML

Juice and blend:

3 tomatoes

2 stalks of celery

5fl oz/145ml still water

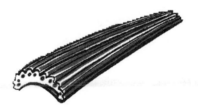

Curly Kale

MAKES APPROX. 10FL OZ/300ML

Juice and blend:

3oz/75g chunk of kale

2 large carrots

5fl oz/145ml still water

Super Carrot

MAKES APPROX. 10FL OZ/300ML
Juice and blend:
1 large carrot
1 stalk of celery
¼ cucumber
5fl oz/145ml still water

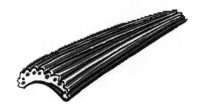

Mango Carrot

MAKES APPROX. 10FL OZ/300ML
Juice and blend:
1 carrot
1 mango (I prefer organic mangoes, they seem to be riper and more juicy)
5fl oz/145ml still water

Happy Apple

MAKES APPROX. 10FL OZ/300ML
Juice and blend:
1 apple
3oz/75g chunk of kale
5fl oz/145ml still water

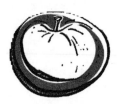

Avocado Smoothie

MAKES APPROX. 10FL OZ/300ML
Juice and blend:
1 large carrot
¼ cucumber
1 avocado, mashed
4fl oz/115ml still water

THE LIFE AND SOUL

Fresh juices can be a delicious addition to a range of party cocktails and punches. Some of them contain alcohol, some are just as delicious without. Give your guests a treat.

Cocktail Kit

- A selection of glasses: short tumbler, tall tumbler (highball), Martini glass, wine glass, large goblet, champagne flute.
- Ice cubes and crushed ice are used in most of the cocktails. To create crushed ice, put some ice cubes in a tea-towel and tie up. Then roll over them with a rolling pin, or give them a bash – they'll soon break up.
- Cocktail shaker and a blender. If you don't have either, put the cocktail into a screw-top jar and shake/blend.
- Swizzle sticks, cocktail umbrellas, cocktail sticks, for decoration.
- Saucer of white sugar for sugar-frosting. Simply rub the rim of the chosen glass with a piece of fruit, then dip into sugar. Sugar will stay on much better using fruit to moisten the rim than if you just use water.
- Cranberry juice is used in quite a few of the recipes; if fresh cranberries are not available, cheat and buy a carton from a shop. It really is a perfect cocktail juice.

Non-Alcoholic Cocktails

Peaches 'n' Cream

SERVES 1

1 peach
1 small orange
6 fresh raspberries
1fl oz/25ml cream
scoop of crushed ice

Juice the peach and orange, blend with the raspberries, cream and crushed ice for 10 seconds. Serve in a tumbler.

Sweet Dreams

SERVES 1
5oz/150g cranberries (or 2fl oz/50ml juice from carton)
3 lychees
dash of grenadine
6 ice cubes

Juice the cranberries with the lychee flesh. Put into a cocktail shaker along with the day of grenadine and the ice cubes. Shake, then drain the cocktail from the ice into a Martini glass.

Sitting Pretty

SERVES 1
2 apricots
1 thick slice of pineapple
½ medium orange
scoop of crushed ice

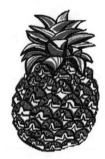

Juice the apricots, pineapple and orange. Blend with crushed ice. Serve in a tall tumbler.

Typhoon

SERVES 1
1 mango
½ medium orange
3oz/75g cranberries (or 1½fl oz/50ml carton juice)
6 ice cubes

Juice the mango, orange and cranberries. Shake together with ice cubes. Pour the whole drink into a tall tumbler.

Honey Bee

SERVES 1
2 peaches
2 tbsps/30ml Greek yoghurt
2fl oz/50ml milk
1 tsp/5ml clear honey

Juice 1½ peaches. Blend with the flesh of the remaining ½ peach, Greek yoghurt, milk and honey. Pour into a tall tumbler.

Grapeberry

SERVES 1
½ grapefruit
7oz/200g cranberries
dash of grenadine
6 ice cubes

Juice the grapefruit and cranberries. Pour into a shaker and add a dash of grenadine and the ice cubes. Shake and strain the liquid off the ice into a wine glass.

Pina Colada

SERVES 1
½ medium pineapple
2 tbsps/30ml coconut cream
1 scoop crushed ice

Juice the pineapple. Blend with the coconut cream and scoop of ice. Serve in a tall tumbler.

Mississippi Mule

SERVES 1
1½ lemons
1½fl oz/35ml cassis
6 ice cubes

Juice the lemons, add the cassis and pour into a shaker with the ice cubes. Shake, then drain the liquid off from the ice cubes and pour into a sugar-frosted Martini glass (see page 153 for how to sugar-frost).

Virgin Mary

SERVES 1
3 tomatoes
squeeze of lemon juice
dash of Tabasco
dash of Worcester sauce
dash of celery salt
freshly ground black pepper
6 ice cubes
stick of celery (for decoration)

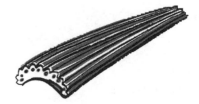

Juice the tomatoes. Pour into a shaker with the lemon juice, Tabasco, Worcester sauce, celery salt, freshly ground black pepper and ice cubes. Shake, then pour the contents into a tall tumbler. Decorate with a stick of celery.

Strawberry Daiquiri

SERVES 1

¼ medium orange

1 lime

6 strawberries

1tsp/5ml clear honey

scoop of crushed ice

Juice the orange and lime. Blend with the strawberries, honey and ice. Serve in a tall tumbler.

Fire Eater

SERVES 1

1 carrot

¼ medium orange

½fl oz/15ml cream

dash of Tabasco

6 ice cubes

Juice the carrot and orange. Pour into a shaker and add the cream, Tabasco and ice. Shake, then drain the liquid off the ice and serve in a wine glass.

Joe Cool

SERVES 1

½ cucumber

dash of salt

squeeze of lemon juice

6 ice cubes

Juice the cucumber. Pour into a shaker and add the salt, lemon juice and ice. Shake, then pour contents into a tall tumbler and top up with soda.

Sweetness and Light

SERVES 1

¼ cucumber

½ medium pineapple

½ avocado, mashed

scoop of crushed ice

10fl oz/300ml lemonade

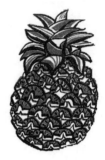

Juice the cucumber and pineapple. Blend with the avocado and ice. Pour into a tall tumbler and top up with lemonade.

Greensleeves

SERVES 1

2 kiwi fruit

1 medium apple

scoop of crushed ice

Juice the kiwi fruit and apple. Blend with the ice. Serve in a tumbler.

Kudos Special

SERVES 1

1 passion fruit

¼ peach

¼ medium orange

½ lemon

6 ice cubes

Juice the passion fruit, peach, orange and lemon. Pour into a shaker with the ice. Shake, and serve in tall tumbler.

Belle des Poires

SERVES 1
1 pear
2 thick slices pineapple
dash of almond syrup

Juice the pear and pineapple. Blend with the almond syrup and serve in a Martini glass.

Redhead

SERVES 1
1 large carrot
2 tomatoes
½ lime
dash of Tabasco
1 tbsp Greek yoghurt
scoop of crushed ice

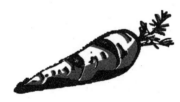

Juice the carrot, tomatoes and lime. Pour into a shaker with the Tabasco, yoghurt and ice. Blend and serve in a tall tumbler.

Bartender's Breakfast

SERVES 1
½ medium orange
1 banana, mashed
4fl oz/115ml milk
1 tsp/5ml clear honey
scoop of crushed ice

Juice the orange. Blend with the banana, milk, honey and ice. Serve in a big goblet.

Strawberry Fields

SERVES 1
1 peach
1 thick slice of pineapple
1 passion fruit
scoop of strawberry ice-cream

Juice the peach, pineapple and passion fruit. Blend with the ice-cream. Serve in large goblet.

Alcoholic Cocktails

Paul's Mai Tai

SERVES 1
¼ medium orange
1 thin slice of pineapple
½ lime
½fl oz/15ml tequila
½fl oz/15ml white rum
½fl oz/15ml dark rum
½fl oz/15ml orange curacao
1fl oz/25ml apricot brandy
dash of Angostura Bitters
dash of almond syrup
dash of grenadine
scoop of crushed ice

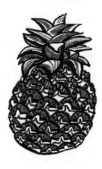

Juice the orange, pineapple and lime. Pour into a shaker and add the tequila, white rum, dark rum, orange curacao, apricot brandy, Angostura bitters, almond syrup, grenadine and ice. Shake and serve in a large goblet.

Orange Blossom

SERVES 1
1 medium orange
2fl oz/50ml gin
6 ice cubes

Juice the orange. Pour into a shaker with the gin. Shake and pour over ice cubes in tall tumbler.

Blondie

SERVES 1
¼ medium orange
½ peach
1fl oz/25ml vodka
½fl oz/15ml peach schnappes
½fl oz/15ml peach liqueur
6 ice cubes

Juice the orange and peach. Pour into a shaker, together with the vodka, peach schnappes, peach liqueur and ice. Shake, then pour into a tall tumbler with sugar-frosted rim (see page 153 for how to sugar-frost).

Peach Daiquiri

SERVES 1

1 lime
1 peach
1fl oz/25ml white rum
1fl oz/25ml peach brandy
½ tsp/5ml clear honey
scoop of crushed ice

Juice the lime and half the peach. Blend with the remaining peach flesh, rum, brandy, honey and ice. Serve in a tall tumbler.

Banana Daiquiri

SERVES 1

1 lime
½ banana, mashed
1fl oz/25ml white rum
1fl oz/25ml banana liqueur
½ tsp/5ml clear honey
scoop of crushed ice

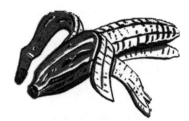

Juice the lime. Blend with the banana, rum, banana liqueur, clear honey and ice. Serve in a tall tumbler.

Planter's Punch

SERVES 1

1 thick slice of pineapple
1 lime
6 ice cubes
2fl oz/50ml golden rum

dash of triple sec/cointreau

dash of grenadine

5fl oz/145ml lemonade

2 slices of orange

2 slices of lemon

Juice the pineapple and lime. Pour over ice in tall tumbler. Add the rum, triple sec/
cointreau, grenadine and top up with lemonade. Stir before drinking. Decorate with the
orange and lemon slices.

Ritz Fizz

SERVES 1

1 lemon

$\frac{1}{2}$fl oz/25ml blue curacao

$\frac{1}{2}$fl oz/25ml amaretto

small bottle of chilled champagne

Juice the lemon. Pour into a champagne flute and add the blue curacao, amaretto, and
top up with champagne.

PUNCHES

Warrior Punch

SERVES 6

8 oranges

1$\frac{1}{2}$lb/700g strawberries

1fl oz/25ml strawberry syrup

3fl oz/80ml strawberry liqueur

3fl oz/80ml melon liqueur

3fl oz/80ml gin

30 ice cubes

Juice the oranges and one third of the strawberries, and pour into a punch bowl. Blend the remaining strawberries into a purée and stir into the orange and strawberry juice. Then add the syrup, the two liqueurs, gin and ice. Serve in punch cups.

Boston Blue Punch

SERVES 6
5 lemons
4fl oz/115ml blue curacao
3fl oz/80ml vodka
3fl oz/80ml gin
2½ pints/1.4 litres chilled lemonade
30 ice cubes

Juice the lemons and pour the liquid into punch bowl. Add the blue curacao, vodka, gin and lemonade. Stir in the ice cubes.

Orange Punch

SERVES 6
10 oranges
3 mangoes
4fl oz/115ml light rum
4fl oz/115ml gold rum
4fl oz/115ml apricot brandy
2½ pints/1.4 litres soda water
30 ice cubes

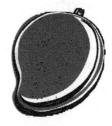

Juice the oranges and mangoes. Pour into a punch bowl. Add the light rum, gold rum, apricot brandy, soda water and ice cubes. Stir and serve.

Exotic Fruit Punch

SERVES 6

2 large pineapples

4 mangoes

4 guavas

4 passion fruit

2 papaya

1lb/450g cranberries

2 pints/1.1 litre lemonade

30 ice cubes

1 star fruit

Juice the pineapples, mangoes, guavas, passion fruit, papayas and cranberries. Pour into a punch bowl. Add the lemonade and ice cubes. Stir. Cut up the star fruit and float star shapes on top of the punch.

Berry Punch

SERVES 6

12 oranges

5oz/150g puréed raspberries

5oz/150g puréed blackberries

5oz/150g puréed strawberries

3 bananas, mashed

2 pints/1.1 litres soda water

30 ice cubes

Juice the oranges and pour into a punch bowl. Stir in the puréed fruits, bananas, soda water and ice cubes. Serve.

pulper's paradise

Every time you make a juice, there will be pulp left over. This is the more fibrous, solid part of the fruit or vegetable that is separated out from the liquid by your juicer. Pulp is not waste, it is a valuable leftover and can be used in all sorts of delicious recipes.

Most mass-market juicers produce pulp that is moist and soft, and therefore easy to combine with other ingredients. It can add extra spice, tang or sweetness to a variety of meals, and is a rich source of fibre. Once you've tried out a few of the recipes in this chapter, you can adapt your own favourite dishes to include pulp – anything from orange to carrot to pineapple. Don't forget, if it pulps, you can cook it!

Ready Reckoner for Pulp

Approximate quantities of pulp produced from fruit and vegetables:

1 lemon	$1^1/4$oz/35g pulp
1 lime	$^1/2$oz/15g pulp
1 orange	2oz/50g pulp
8oz/225g carrots	$4^1/4$oz/120g pulp
6 tomatoes	$3^1/2$oz/90g pulp
1 mango	$2^1/2$oz/65g pulp
15 large spinach leaves	$1^1/4$oz/35g pulp
8oz/225g pineapple	4oz/125g pulp
8 plums	4oz/125g pulp
6 sticks celery	2oz/50g pulp
4 eating apples	$2^3/4$oz/70g pulp
4 peaches	2oz/50g pulp

carrot and orange soup

serves 4

1 Melt the margarine in a pan. Add the onion and carrots and stir. Cook gently for 5 minutes.
2 Stir in the remaining ingredients, cover the pan and cook gently for 30 minutes, until the carrots are soft.
3 Allow the soup to cool slightly. Purée in a blender or food processor.
4 Return to the pan and reheat gently. Serve garnished with coriander (cilantro).

1oz/15g sunflower margarine
1 onion, peeled and finely chopped
1lb/450g carrots, thinly sliced
1¼ pints/750ml vegetable or chicken stock
1 tbsp/15ml fresh coriander (cilantro)
1 orange, juice and pulp
sea salt
freshly ground black pepper
chopped fresh coriander (cilantro) to garnish

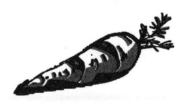

spicy spinach pâté

serves 4–6

1tbsp/15ml olive oil
1 onion, peeled and finely chopped
1 clove garlic, crushed
8oz/225g carrots, coarsely grated
pulp from 15 large spinach leaves
6tbsp/90ml plain fromage frais
2oz/50g/1 cup wholewheat breadcrumbs
1 egg, beaten
1tbsp/15ml fresh lemon juice
1tsp/5ml ground allspice
few drops of Tabasco sauce
sea salt
freshly ground black pepper

1 Heat the olive oil in a pan. Fry the onion and garlic for 2 minutes. Add the carrots and cook for 5 minutes.
2 Remove the pan from the heat and add all the remaining ingredients, mixing thoroughly.
3 Spoon the mixture into a greased 1lb/450g loaf tin and level the surface.
4 Bake in a pre-heated oven at 180°C/350°F/Gas Mark 4 for 35–40 minutes, until golden brown.
5 Leave to cool in the tin and then turn out and refrigerate until ready to serve.
6 Serve hot or cold, with a green salad.

mango chicken

serves 4

1   Brush the chicken breasts with the oil and season with salt and pepper. Grill (broil) under a medium heat for about 20 minutes, turning occasionally, until thoroughly cooked through. Set aside and keep warm.

2   Melt the margarine in a pan. Stir in the flour and cook gently for 1 minute.

3   Remove the pan from the heat and gradually stir in the milk. Bring to the boil slowly and continue to cook, stirring all the time, until the sauce thickens. Simmer gently for 5 minutes.

4   Add the mango juice and pulp, ginger, garlic, salt and black pepper and mix well. Simmer for 2 minutes.

5   Serve the chicken breasts with the sauce poured over them.

4 chicken breasts
1tbsp/15ml sunflower oil
sea salt
freshy ground black pepper
$1^{1}/_2$oz/40g sunflower margarine
2oz/50g/1 cup plain flour
$^{3}/_4$ pint/450ml/2 cups semi-skimmed milk
1 mango, juice and pulp
(I prefer organic mangoes, they seem to be riper and more juicy)
1 piece fresh ginger
(approx. $^{1}/_2$ inch/1.5cm square), peeled and finely chopped
1 clove garlic, crushed

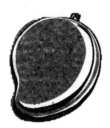

nutty stuffed peppers

serves 4

4 large (bell) peppers, red, yellow or green

1oz/25g sunflower margarine

1 onion, finely chopped

2oz/50g/$\frac{1}{2}$ cup Cheddar cheese, grated

2oz/50g/$\frac{1}{2}$ cup (English) walnuts, roughly chopped

1 clove garlic, crushed

2oz/50g/1 cup wholewheat breadcrumbs

pulp from 6 tomatoes

3tbsp/45ml fresh tomato juice

4tbsp/60ml fresh parsley, finely chopped

sea salt

freshly ground black pepper

1 Slice the 'lids' off the (bell) peppers and remove cores and seeds. Blanch in boiling water for 5 minutes. Drain.

2 Melt the margarine in a pan. Add the onion and cook for 3 minutes.

3 Remove the pan from the heat. Add all the remaining ingredients and mix well.

4 Place the mixture inside the (bell) peppers and replace the 'lids'.

5 Place the stuffed (bell) peppers in a deep oven-proof dish which has a little water in the bottom. Cover with foil and bake in a pre-heated oven at 180°C/350°F/ Gas Mark 4, for 35–40 minutes.

6 Serve hot with a selection of fresh vegetables or with warm French bread.

herby carrot burgers

serves 6

1 Place all the ingredients in a bowl and mix well to combine.
2 Form the mixture into 6 burgers and brush each one with a little oil.
3 Grill (broil) the burgers under a medium heat for 15–20 minutes, turning once.
4 Serve with a brown rice salad.

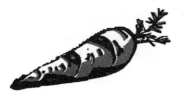

12oz/350g/1^{1}/2 cups lean minced beef
1 onion, peeled and finely chopped
4oz/125g carrots, coarsely grated
pulp from 12oz/350g carrots
4oz/125g/1 cup Cheddar cheese, grated
4oz/125g/1 cup wheatgerm
1 egg, beaten
2tbsp/30ml fresh parsley, finely chopped
2tbsp/30ml fresh thyme, finely chopped
sea salt
freshly ground black pepper
vegetable oil for brushing

spicy vegetable couscous

serves 6

1lb/450g/4 cups couscous
2 onions, finely chopped
3 courgettes (zucchini), sliced
8oz/225g cauliflower, broken into florets
1 green (bell) pepper, de-seeded and cut into thin strips
4oz/125g/1 cup white cabbage, shredded
3 tomatoes, skinned and chopped
3 carrots, sliced
pulp from 8oz/225g carrots
2 sticks celery, sliced
pulp from 6 sticks celery
1 14oz/400g tin kidney beans, rinsed and drained
2 pints/1.1 litres vegetable stock
2 cloves garlic, crushed
2tbsp/30ml fresh coriander (cilantro), finely chopped
pinch of cayenne pepper
2tsp/10ml ground cumin
$^{1}/_{2}$tsp/2.5ml saffron threads
2tbsp/30ml olive oil

1 Put the couscous in a large bowl with ¾ pint/450ml of tepid water and leave to soak for 1 hour.
2 Place the prepared vegetables and pulp in a large saucepan with the stock, garlic, coriander (cilantro), spices and saffron. Bring to the boil, cover and simmer for 30 minutes.
3 Drain the couscous and put in a steamer over the saucepan of vegetables. Cover and continue cooking for a further 40 minutes, then remove steamer and cover saucepan, keeping the vegetables simmering.
4 Place the couscous in a large mixing bowl. Beat the oil into the couscous with 2tbsp/30ml of lightly salted water. Leave to stand for 10 minutes.
5 Stir the couscous to remove any lumps and return to the steamer over the simmering vegetables for 20 minutes, covered.
6 Season the vegetables and serve with the couscous on a warmed serving dish.

prawn and mango filo parcels

serves 6

1 Place the prawns, spring onions (scallions), garlic, mango pulp, cumin and seasoning in a bowl and mix well.

2 To make the filo parcels, brush each pastry sheet with melted margarine and cut out three 4 inch/10cm squares. Pile the three squares on top of each other and add some of the filling mixture. Gather up the corners to enclose the filling and twist to seal. Repeat for each parcel, and brush each one with melted margarine. Place the parcels on a greased baking tray.

3 Bake in a pre-heated oven at 200°C/400°F/Gas Mark 6, until golden brown.

4 Serve with a green salad or fresh vegetables.

12oz/350g peeled prawns
4 spring onions (scallions), finely chopped
1 clove garlic, crushed
pulp from 2 medium mangoes
1tsp/5ml ground cumin
sea salt
freshly ground black pepper
6 sheets of filo pastry
2oz/50g melted vegetable margarine

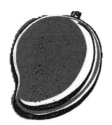

red wine spaghetti

serves 4–6

1½lb/700g ripe tomatoes
1tbsp/15ml olive oil
1 medium onion, sliced
2–3 cloves garlic, crushed
2tbsp/30ml dried basil
pinch of salt
freshly ground black pepper,
to taste
1tbsp/15ml tomato paste
1tbsp/15ml red wine
3oz/75g pine kernels
1lb/450g long spaghetti
4oz/125g Parmesan cheese
(optional)

1 Juice ½lb/225g of tomatoes, set juice and pulp aside. Chop up the remaining tomatoes into small chunks and gently fry in some of the olive oil.

2 Heat up the remaining olive oil in a separate pan and gently fry the sliced onion. After five minutes add the crushed garlic, chopped tomatoes, dried basil and salt and pepper. Fry for a further five minutes.

3 Add the tomato juice and pulp, tomato paste, red wine and pine kernels. Simmer for half an hour.

4 Ten minutes before cooking time has elapsed, bring a large saucepan of slightly salted water to the boil. Add in spaghetti and cook until *al dente* (firm to the bite – but not undercooked).

5 When spaghetti is cooked, drain and place in a large bowl. Pour red wine sauce over the top. Sprinkle with Parmesan cheese, if using, and serve with a crisp green salad.

sweet and sour pork

serves 4–6

1 Heat the oil in a large frying pan (skillet) or wok. Add the pork and cook until brown all over (about 5 or 10 minutes).

2 Add the vegetables and nuts and stir-fry for 8–10 minutes, until cooked through.

3 Combine all the remaining ingredients and add to the pork mixture. Stir-fry for a couple of minutes and thicken with cornflour (cornstarch) if desired.

4 Serve immediately with brown rice or noodles.

5 Add sea salt and freshly ground black pepper to taste.

1tbsp/15ml sesame oil
1lb/450g pork fillet, cut into
1 inch/2.5cm strips
4oz/125g/1$^{1}/_{2}$ cups
mushrooms, sliced
8 spring onions (scallions),
finely chopped
4oz/125g beansprouts
1 8oz/225g tin (can) of
bamboo shoots, drained
6oz/175g mangetout
(snow peas)
6oz/175g courgettes
(zucchini), sliced thinly
1 clove garlic, crushed
4oz/125g cashew nuts
1tbsp/15ml clear honey
1tbsp/15ml soy sauce
$^{1}/_{4}$ pint/150ml vegetable
stock
2tbsp/30ml cider vinegar
pulp from 6oz/175g
pineapple
pulp from 1 lime
pulp from 3 plums
cornflour (cornstarch) to
thicken (optional)

chilli bean pot

serves 4

1lb/450g ripe tomatoes
2 large sticks celery
1/2 large lemon
8oz/225g tinned (canned)
kidney beans
4oz/125g tinned (canned)
blackeye beans
4oz/125g tinned (canned)
butter beans
4oz/125g mushrooms, sliced
2tbsp/30ml fresh oregano
1–2tsp/5–10ml chilli
powder, or one fresh chilli,
chopped

1 Juice the tomatoes, celery and lemon, and place pulp and juice in a large casserole dish. Drain beans.

2 Add all the other ingredients and stir. Place in the oven at 190°C/375°F/Gas Mark 5 for 40 minutes, stirring occasionally. Serve straight to table in the casserole dish, with brown rice.

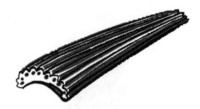

pasta with bacon and celery

serves 4–6

1 Cook the pasta in a large pan of lightly salted boiling water, for 8–10 minutes, or until *al dente*. Drain well.
2 Meanwhile, grill (broil) the bacon until crisp, then cut into small bite-sized pieces.
3 Combine the remaining ingredients, add the hot pasta and bacon, mix well and serve either hot or cold.

12oz/350g wholewheat pasta shapes
4oz/125g smoked back bacon rashers
6oz/175g/1^1/2 cups Cheddar cheese, grated
4oz/125g/1^1/2 cups mushrooms, sliced
4 celery sticks, thinly sliced
pulp from 6 sticks celery
3 medium tomatoes, chopped
pulp from 6 tomatoes
1tbsp/15ml fresh parsley, finely chopped
1tbsp/15ml fresh chives, finely chopped
sea salt
freshly ground black pepper

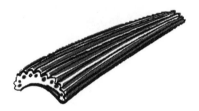

lemon chicken and sesame stir-fry

serves 4–6

6tbsp/90ml chicken stock
2tsp/10ml sherry
2tsp/10ml soy sauce
1tsp/5ml soft brown sugar
1 clove garlic, crushed
juice and pulp from 1 lemon
2tbsp/30ml fresh tarragon,
finely chopped
sea salt
freshly ground black pepper
1lb/450g chicken breasts,
cut into 1 inch/2.5cm strips
1tbsp/15ml sesame oil
1 leek, thinly sliced
6oz/175g carrots, cut into
thin strips
4oz/125g mangetout
(snow peas)
1 7oz/200g tin (can)
sweetcorn, drained
1oz/25g sesame seeds
cornflour (cornstarch) to
thicken (optional)

1 Mix together the stock, sherry, soy sauce, sugar, garlic, lemon juice and pulp, tarragon and seasoning. Add the chicken, stir well and leave to marinade in the refrigerator for a couple of hours.

2 Heat the oil in a large frying pan (skillet) or wok. Stir-fry the chicken until cooked. Add the vegetables and sesame seeds and stir-fry until just cooked through, mixing well. Thicken the sauce with cornflour (cornstarch), if desired.

3 Serve immediately with brown rice or noodles.

thai-style fish casserole

1   Heat the oil in a large flameproof casserole. Add the spring onions (scallions) and (bell) peppers and fry for 3 minutes.
2   Add the tomatoes, fruit pulp, soy sauce, ginger, sherry and seasoning, mix well and gently bring to the boil. Simmer for 5 minutes.
3   Remove from heat. Lay the cod fillets on top of the vegetable mixture, cover and cook in a pre-heated oven at 180°C/350°F/Gas Mark 4, for 30 minutes, until the fish is cooked.
4   Sprinkle with chopped parsley and serve immediately with boiled new potatoes.

1tbsp/15ml olive oil
6 spring onions (scallions), finely chopped
1 green (bell) pepper, de-seeded and cut into thin strips
1 red (bell) pepper, de-seeded and cut into thin strips
1 14oz/400g tin (can) chopped tomatoes with herbs
pulp from 1 lemon
pulp from 1 lime
pulp from 4 plums
2tsp/10ml soy sauce
1 piece of fresh ginger, approx. 1 inch/2.5cm square, peeled and finely chopped
2 tbsp/30ml sherry
sea salt
freshly ground black pepper
4 cod fillets
2tbsp/30ml fresh parsley, finely chopped, to garnish

crispy red cabbage and apple salad

serves 4

1 small red cabbage, finely shredded
2 green-skinned eating apples, cored and sliced
6oz/175g/1 cup sultanas (golden seedless raisins)
pulp from 4 eating apples
2tbsp/30ml fresh apple juice
$1/4$ pint/150ml/$2/3$ cup plain yoghurt
1tbsp/15ml olive oil
sea salt
freshly ground black pepper

1 Place all the ingredients in a large bowl and mix well to combine.

2 Serve the salad on its own or as an accompaniment to pasta or rice dishes.

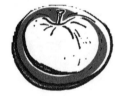

brown rice salad

1 Cook the rice in a large pan of salted boiling water,
   for 15–20 minutes, until tender. Rinse, drain and cool.
2 Beat together the oil, vinegar, garlic and thyme to
   make a dressing.
3 Place all the remaining ingredients in a large bowl,
   add the rice and oil dressing and mix thoroughly.
4 Leave to stand for 30 minutes and then serve.

8oz/225g/1$\frac{1}{2}$ cups long
grain brown rice
4tbsp/60ml olive oil
2tbsp/30ml cider vinegar
1 clove garlic, crushed
1tbsp/15ml fresh thyme,
finely chopped
3oz/75g/^{3}/$_4$ cup red
Leicester cheese, grated
6oz/175g/2 cups mush-
rooms, sliced
8 spring onions (scallions),
finely chopped
2 celery sticks, thinly sliced
pulp from 8oz/225g
pineapple
pulp from 4 peaches
sea salt
freshly ground black pepper

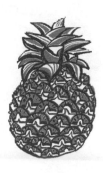

mixed fruit and
vegetable salad

serves 4

3oz/75g alfalfa sprouts or
two cartons mustard
and cress
4 celery sticks, thinly sliced
2 medium bananas, peeled
and sliced
1 large carrot, coarsely
grated
4oz/125g/2 cup raisins
2oz/50g/^{1}/2 cup hazelnuts,
roughly chopped
3tbsp/45ml Greek yoghurt
pulp from 1 orange
pulp from 8oz/225g
pineapple
2tbsp/30ml fresh pineapple
juice
sea salt
freshly ground black pepper

1 Place all the ingredients in a large bowl and mix well
to combine.
2 Serve the salad on its own, with pasta or rice, or as an
accompaniment to meat.

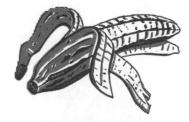

tangy lemon and lime mousse

serves 4–6

1 Sprinkle the gelatine over the fruit juices in a small bowl and leave to soak. Place the bowl over a saucepan of simmering water, and stir until the gelatine has dissolved. Leave to cool slightly.

2 Mix together the grated fruit rind, fruit pulp, honey and fromage frais in a bowl. Stir in the gelatine mixture and mix well.

3 Whisk the egg whites until stiff, and fold gently into the mixture.

4 Gently put the mixture into a shallow dish or individual ramekins, then chill in the refrigerator until set. Garnish with mint leaves.

1tbsp/15ml gelatine
grated rind, juice and pulp of 1 lemon
grated rind, juice and pulp of 1 lime
3tbsp/45ml thick honey
$^3/_4$ pint/450ml/2 cups plain fromage frais
2 egg whites
mint leaves to garnish

mixed berry crumble

serves 4

8oz/225g/2 cups blackcurrants	1 Put the blackcurrants and raspberries in a pan with 2tbsp/30ml water and cook gently until just softened. Remove from the heat and stir in the lemon and orange pulp and 2oz/50g of the brown sugar.
8oz/225g/2$\frac{1}{2}$ cups raspberries	
pulp from 1 lemon	2 Put the fruit mixture into a 2 pint/1.1 litre dish.
pulp from 1 orange	3 Melt the margarine in a saucepan. Remove from heat and stir in the remaining sugar, oats and mixed spice. Mix well.
4oz/125g/1 cup soft brown sugar	
2oz/50g sunflower margarine	4 Spoon the crumble mixture over the fruit and press down lightly.
4oz/125g/1 cup rolled oats	5 Bake in a pre-heated oven at 180°C/350°F/ Gas Mark 4 for 30 minutes, until the crumble is golden brown and crisp.
1tsp/5ml mixed spice	
	6 Serve hot or cold with fromage frais or custard.

wholewheat crêpes
with peach sauce

serves 4

To make the crêpes

1 Sift the flour and salt into a bowl and make a well in
the centre. Add the egg and beat well with a wooden
spoon. Gradually beat in the milk to make a smooth
batter.

2 Heat a little oil in a 7inch/18cm frying pan (skillet),
until hot. Pour off any surplus; there should be just
enough to cover the surface.

3 Pour in just enough batter to coat thinly the base of
the pan. Cook for 1–2 minutes, until golden brown,
turn and cook the second side until golden.

4 Transfer the crêpe to a plate and keep hot.

5 Repeat with the remaining batter to make 8 crêpes.
Pile the cooked crêpes on top of each other with
greaseproof (waxed) paper between each one and put
aside to keep warm.

To make the sauce

1 Mix the cornflour (cornstarch) with 2tbsp/30ml of
the water, stir until dissolved.

2 Add the rest of the water and the remaining
ingredients, mixing well.

3 Bring gently to the boil, stirring continuously, then
simmer for 3 minutes.

4 Serve the hot crêpes with the peach sauce poured over
each one.

For the crêpes

4oz/125g/1 cup wholewheat
flour
pinch of salt
1 egg, beaten
$1/2$ pint/300ml/$1^1/4$ cups
semi-skimmed milk
vegetable oil for frying

For the peach sauce

5tsp/25ml cornflour
(cornstarch)
$1/2$ pint/300ml/$1^1/4$ cups
cold water
2oz/50g/$1/2$ cup soft brown
sugar
3 peaches, peeled and finely
chopped
pulp from 4 peaches
2tbsp/30ml fresh peach
juice
1tsp/5ml ground nutmeg

peach and banana brûlée

serves 6

1 pint/600ml/2¹/₂ cups
double (heavy) cream
4 egg yolks
4oz/125g/¹/₂ cup
caster sugar
pulp from 4 peaches
2 small bananas

1   Pour the cream into a mixing bowl placed over a pan of simmering water. Warm gently until almost boiling, then remove from the heat.

2   Beat together the egg yolks and 2oz/50g/¹/₄ cup of the sugar until light in colour. Gradually pour on the cream, whisking gently until evenly mixed. Mix in the peach pulp.

3   Stand 6 ramekins in a roasting dish, with about ¹/₂ inch/1cm water around the bases of the ramekins.

4   Peel and slice the bananas and place several slices in the base of each ramekin.

5   Pour the custard mixture slowly into the ramekins, dividing it equally between them.

6   Bake in a pre-heated oven at 150°C/300°F/ Gas Mark 2, for about 1 hour, or until set. Remove from the tin and leave to cool, then refrigerate overnight.

7   Sprinkle the remaining sugar evenly over the top of each brûlée and put under a hot grill (broiler) for 2–3 minutes until the sugar turns to caramel. Leave to cool, then chill before serving.

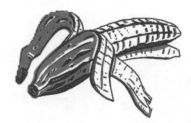

berry yoghurt

**makes 1¹⁄₂ pints/
850ml**

1 Bring the milk to the boil, then reduce heat and
   simmer for one minute. Then let cool.
2 As the milk cools, whip up the yoghurt in a bowl.
   When the milk has become tepid, gradually add it to
   the yoghurt and whisk in.
3 Add in the berry pulp, then cover the bowl with the
   clingfilm, and leave to set for around 8 hours.
4 Once the yoghurt has set, refrigerate.

1¹⁄₂ pints/900ml/4 cups milk
2tbsp/30ml plain yoghurt
pulp of 6oz/175g/2 cups
strawberries
pulp of 6oz/175g/2 cups
raspberries
pulp of 6oz/175g/2 cups
blackberries

orange and raspberry sherbet

serves 4

1lb/450g/4 cups raspberries
2 large oranges
2tbsp/30ml honey

1 Juice the raspberries and the oranges. Place pulp and juice in a bowl and stir in the honey.

2 Pour the mixture into a shallow dish, and freeze until almost firm. Then remove from the dish, break up and mix until fluffy.

3 Pour the mixture back into the dish and freeze until firm.

4 Remove dish from freezer 15 minutes before serving, so that it thaws slightly. Then scoop and serve.

carrot and banana cake

serves 6

1 Grease a 7 inch/18cm diameter round cake tin and line with greaseproof (wax) paper.
2 Sift the flour into a bowl. Stir in the remaining ingredients and beat together until well mixed.
3 Spoon the mixture into the tin and level the surface.
4 Bake in a pre-heated oven at 150°C/300°F/Gas Mark 2 for 1½ hours, until well-risen and golden brown.
5 Cool in the tin for 30 minutes, then turn out and cool on a wire rack.

8oz/225g/2 cups self-raising wholewheat flour
5oz/150g/1 cup soft brown sugar
¼ pint/150ml/½ cup sunflower oil
2 eggs, beaten
2 large bananas, peeled and mashed
5oz/150g carrots, coarsely grated
pulp from 8oz/225g carrots
1oz/25g/¼ cup (English) walnuts, chopped

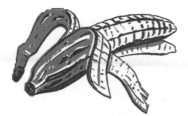

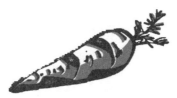

apricot, nut and plum teabread

serves 6

4oz/125g/^{1}/2 cup dried apricots, roughly chopped

3oz/75g/^{3}/4 cup bran

^{1}/2 pint/300ml/1^1/4 cups semi-skimmed milk

6oz/175g/1^1/2 cups self-raising wholewheat flour

2oz/50g/^{1}/2 cup mixed nuts, chopped

3oz/75g/^{3}/4 cup soft brown sugar

1 egg, beaten

pulp from 8 plums

1 Grease a 2lb/900g loaf tin.

2 Soak the apricots and bran in the milk for 5 minutes.

3 Sift the flour into a large bowl, add the bran mixture and all the remaining ingredients and mix well.

4 Turn the mixture into the tin and level the surface.

5 Bake in a pre-heated oven at 190°C/375°F/ Gas Mark 5, for 1–1^1/4 hours, until firm to touch.

6 Turn out and cool on a wire rack. Store for a couple of days before eating (this makes it more moist).

7 Serve slices buttered, with preserves.

1 glossary: vitamins and minerals

Vitamins and minerals are essential to life. We need most of them only in tiny amounts, but they are still vital to our well-being. Although full-blown deficiency diseases are now extremely rare in the Western world, we can still suffer milder symptoms of deficiencies, and it is important to ensure that we consume sufficient quantities of vitamins and minerals to stay in peak health.

Fresh fruit and vegetable juices are excellent natural sources of vitamins and minerals. **The very best source for each particular vitamin/mineral is highlighted.**

VITAMINS

Vitamin A/beta-carotene

Vitamin A is needed to maintain healthy teeth, gums, bones, skin, hair and eyes. It protects the mucous membranes in the body (eg the throat, lungs and digestive system) and helps build up immunity against illness.

Vitamin A (retinol) is only found in animal produce such as dairy foods, liver and eggs. However, the body can also obtain vitamin A from fruit and vegetable sources via another nutrient called beta-carotene. Orange fruit and vegetables and green, leafy vegetables are rich in beta-carotene, which the digestive system is able to convert into vitamin A.

Vitamin A (retinol) and beta-carotene are both antioxidants (see Chapter 1).

Best Fruit Juices
Apricot, mango, melon (orange flesh), nectarine, orange, peach, tangerine.

Best Vegetable Juices
Broccoli, cabbage, **carrot**, kale, lettuce, spinach, watercress, wheatgrass.

Vitamin B Complex

Vitamin B complex is not just one substance: there are over ten members of the vitamin B complex group, so their role is more complex than that of their fellow vitamins and minerals. It's useful to bear in mind that if you smoke, drink, take the contraceptive pill, or are elderly, pregnant or lactating, you may require more of the B complex group than normal (consult your general practitioner if you are in one of these categories and think you may need to take supplements).

On the whole, B vitamins are found more abundantly in vegetables than in fruit. Although avocados and bananas are difficult to juice, they are both high in B vitamins, and can be mashed and blended with other juices. The important vitamin B12 is not found in vegetable or fruit sources, so cannot be consumed through a juice; it is found in eggs and fortified cereals.

Vitamin B1 (Thiamine)

Plays a major role in the production of energy for the body, helping to digest and metabolize foods containing carbohydrate (starch). It also influences the health of the heart, muscles and nervous system. Those on the contraceptive pill and those who smoke or drink heavily may be low in B1.

Best Fruit Juices
Orange, pineapple, plum, **tangerine**.

Best Vegetable Juices
Cauliflower, garlic, **kale**, leek, mangetout (snow pea), parsley.

Vitamin B2 (Riboflavin)

Helps with the release of energy. It also promotes general growth and healthy skin, eyes, mouth, hair and nails.

Best Fruit Juices
Apricot, blackcurrant, **cherry**, kiwi fruit, peach.

Best Vegetable Juices
Bean sprout, broccoli, **kale**, mangetout (snow pea), parsley, red (bell) pepper, spinach, watercress.

Vitamin B3 (Niacin)

Helps form certain enzymes which are used in the conversion and metabolism of energy from food.

Best Fruit Juices

Grape, grapefruit, guava, **passion fruit**, peach, strawberry.

Best Vegetable Juices

Bean sprout, carrot, cauliflower, **kale**, parsley, potato, red (bell) pepper.

Vitamin B5 (Pantothenic acid)

Plays a crucial role in making energy available to the body.

Best Fruit Juices

Blackberry, lemon, raspberry, strawberry, **watermelon**.

Best Vegetable Juices

Broccoli, cauliflower, celery, sweet potato.

Vitamin B6 (Pyridoxine)

Plays a major role in the metabolism of protein, essential body chemicals, sugar and fatty acids. Helps to keep nerves and skin healthy.

Best Fruit Juices

Blackcurrant, **banana**, raspberry, watermelon.

Best Vegetable Juices

Brussels sprout, kale, leek, green (bell) pepper, sweet potato.

Folic Acid

Helps to keep the nervous system healthy. It is also an essential nutrient for pregnant women, as it can prevent the disabling condition spina bifida occurring in babies. Folic acid is found in much larger amounts in vegetables than fruits.

Best Fruit Juices
Melon, orange, pineapple, strawberry, tangerine.

Best Vegetable Juices
Beetroot, broccoli, **Brussels sprout**, cabbage (winter), cauliflower, lettuce (round), parsnip.

Biotin, Choline, Inositol

These are lesser known, but equally important B vitamins which are found in very small quantities in green, leafy vegetables.

Vitamin C

Vitamin C plays an important role in the production of collagen, the connective tissue found in skin and bones. As a 'skin' vitamin it can accelerate wound healing, and is a powerful antioxidant which protects against some degenerative diseases (see Chapter 1). It also facilitates the absorption of iron. The body uses up vitamin C more rapidly if you are under stress, if you smoke or are taking antibiotics. Vitamin C is found abundantly in both fruits and vegetables. The majority of fruits contain vitamin C; those listed below are the richest.

Best Fruit Juices
Blackberry, **blackcurrant**, blueberry, gooseberry, grapefruit, guava, kiwi fruit, lemon, lime, mango, melon, orange, papaya, pineapple, raspberry, strawberry, tangerine.

Best Vegetable Juices

Broccoli, Brussels sprout, cabbage (red, white, winter), cauliflower, fennel, **parsley**, green (bell) pepper, watercress.

Vitamin E

Vitamin E is a powerful antioxidant and helps protect the body from the damaging effects of free radicals. It also prevents polyunsaturated fats from being oxidized, and supports the work of vitamin A/beta-carotene. It tends to be concentrated in green, leafy vegetables.

Best Fruit Juices

Blackberry, blackcurrant, gooseberry, grapefruit, **grape (white)**, greengage, plum, raspberry.

Best Vegetable Juices

Brussels sprout, cabbage, carrot, celery, leek, lettuce, parsnip, green (bell) pepper, **sweet potato**, spinach, tomato, watercress.

MINERALS

There are nine major minerals that can be found in relatively high levels in fruit and vegetables: calcium, chlorine, iron, magnesium, phosphorus, potassium, sodium, sulphur and zinc. Other minerals found in lesser amounts are chromium, cobalt, copper, fluorine, iodine, manganese and selenium.

Calcium

Essential for strong bones and teeth. It is widely available in both fruits and vegetables.

Best Fruit Juices

Blackberry, blackcurrant, gooseberry, grape, guava, kiwi fruit, papaya, raspberry, strawberry.

Best Vegetable Juices

Broccoli, cabbage (red, savoy, spring, white, winter), carrot, celery, fennel, **kale**, mangetout (snow pea), parsnip, green (bell) pepper, spinach, watercress.

Chlorine

Helps to regulate the body's acid/alkaline balance, and aids the liver in cleaning out waste material.

Best Fruit Juices

Blackberry, blackcurrant, **melon (honeydew and cantaloupe)**, passion fruit, raspberry, strawberry.

Best Vegetable Juices

Brussels sprout, carrot, celery, leek, lettuce (round), sweet potato, **watercress**.

Iron

Essential for the manufacture of red blood corpuscles which transport oxygen around the body. Iron also helps to make certain enzymes. Women lose more iron than men, due to menstruation.

Best Fruit Juices

Blackberry, **blackcurrant**, cranberry, passion fruit, raspberry.

Best Vegetable Juices

Kale, leek, lettuce (cos), mangetout (snow pea), **parsley**, radish, spinach, sweet potato, watercress.

Magnesium

Vital for many enzyme processes, and helps distribute sodium, potassium and calcium throughout cells. Essential for muscle and nerve functioning.

Best Fruit Juices

Blackberry, blackcurrant, grape, grapefruit, guava, kiwi fruit, lemon, melon, **passion fruit**, raspberry, strawberry.

Best Vegetable Juices

Beetroot, **broccoli**, Brussels sprout, cabbage, celeriac, mangetout (snow pea), turnip, parsnip.

Phosphorus

Vital for the majority of chemical reactions in the body. Essential for kidney function, strong teeth and bones.

Best Fruit Juices

Blackcurrant, grape, guava, kiwi fruit, melon, passion fruit, raspberry, strawberry.

Best Vegetable Juices

Alfalfa sprout, broccoli, **celeriac**, kale, parsnip.

Potassium

Found in all our cells, in particular it ensures that the body's water balance and heart rhythm is regulated, and it plays a role in the health of muscles and nerves.

Best Fruit Juices

Apricot, **blackcurrant**, cherry, grape, greengage, guava, kiwi fruit, melon, papaya, passion fruit, peach, raspberry.

Best Vegetable Juices

Beetroot, broccoli, Brussels sprout, cabbage, cauliflower, celeriac, celery, fennel, kale, leek, lettuce, parsnip, radish, **spinach**, tomato, watercress.

Sodium

Needed for the regulation of body fluids and blood pressure. Most of us eat more than enough sodium through our diet, and too much can produce high blood pressure. The amounts found in fruits and vegetables are not likely to be harmful, if your diet is not already over-loaded with salt. The following juices can help to replace sodium lost from the body in cases of heatstroke.

Best Fruit Juices
Blackberry, blackcurrant, cherry, kiwi fruit, lemon, melon, **passion fruit**.

Best Vegetable Juices
Beetroot, broccoli, cabbage, carrot, celeriac, **celery**, kale, radish, spinach, watercress.

Sulphur

Essential for healthy skin, hair and nails. It also aids in metabolic processes in the brain and liver.

Best Fruit Juices
Blackcurrant, gooseberry, grape (white), melon, passion fruit, raspberry, strawberry.

Best Vegetable Juices
Carrot, celery, cucumber, onion, parsnip, radish, sweet potato, tomato, **watercress**.

Zinc

Vital for many processes affecting the body's cells, it helps to build cells, bolsters the immune system, and plays an active role in the health of the reproductive systems of men and women. It also helps balance the body's acid/alkaline content.

Best Fruit Juices
Guava, **raspberry**.

Best Vegetable Juices
Broccoli, **Brussels sprout**, tomato, watercress.

Chromium, Cobalt, Copper, Fluorine, Iodine, Manganese, Selenium

These minerals are found in very small quantities in most fresh fruits, but only in leafy green vegetables. They can be found in abundance in organ meats, seafood, nuts and wholegrains.

2 useful information

PROFESSIONAL ADVICE

United Kingdom

Council for Complementary and Alternative Medicine
Park House
206–208 Latimer Road
London W10 6RE
Tel: 020 8968 3862

British Complementary Medical Association
249 Fosse Road
Leicester LE3 1AE
Tel: 0116 2825511

The Community Health Foundation
188 Old Street
London EC1V 9FR
Tel: 020 7251 4076

General Council and Register of Naturopaths
Goswell House
2 Goswell Road
Street
Somerset BA16 0JG
Tel: 01458 840072

The Internet is also a valuable source of information and help.

United States of America

American Association of Naturopathic Physicians

8201 Greensboro Drive

Suite 300

McLean

Virginia 22102

Tel: 703 610 9037

Fax: 703 610 9005

www.naturopathic.org

American Holistic Medical Association

4101 Lake Boone Trail

Suite 201

Raleigh

North Carolina 27607

Tel: 703 556 9245

www.holisticmedicine.org

National Center for Homeopathy

801 North Fairfax Street

Suite 306

Alexandria

Virginia 22314

Tel: 703 548 7790

www.homeopathic.org

Australia

Natural Health Society of Australia

(A non-profit organization; addresses are subject to change)

New South Wales:

Head Office (047) 215068

Eastern Suburbs (02) 373024

Parramatta (02) 6378609

Pymble (02) 4492741

Sutherland (02) 5259907

www.cetacean.com.au/nhsa

Central Coast (043) 821345

Newcastle (049) 439979

Wollongong (042) 291349

ACT:

Canberra (06) 2317593

Victoria:

Melbourne (03) 8882124

Queensland:

Brisbane (07) 3533283

Cairns (070) 576600

Townsville (077) 231122

Northern Territory:

Darwin (089) 278784

FOODS FOR THE ONE WEEK VITALITY PLAN

Freshlands Wholefoods stocks a wide range of wholegrains, sea vegetables, rice cakes, seeds and lots more. Find them at 196 Old Street, London EC1V 9BP, tel: 020 7250 1708. Freshlands also offers a mail order service on the following telephone number: 020 8746 2261.

Planet Organic stores in London also stock a wide range of dried seeds, pulses and organic fruit and vegetables.

Planet Organic

42 Westbourne Grove
London W2 5SH
Tel: 020 7727 2227
or
22 Torrington Place
London WC1A 7JE
Tel: 020 7436 1929
for mail order call:
020 7221 1345

SPECIALIST EQUIPMENT

Reasonably priced brands of juicer that can be found in high-street stores include Braun, Philips, Kenwood and Moulinex. Before shopping why not look them up on the Internet to check out their various models for capacity, price and look. Find their websites at:

www.braun.com
www.philips.co.uk
www.kenwood.co.uk
www.moulinex.com

A wide variety of specialist juicers and useful juicing aids can be obtained by mail order from the Wholistic Research Company, Bright Haven, Robin's Lane, Lolworth, Cambridge CB3 8HH, tel: 01954 781074.

further reading

Juicing

Blauer, Stephen, *The Juicing Book*, Avery, 1989.

Calbom, Cherie and Maureen B. Keane, *Juicing for Life*, Avery, 1992.

The Complete Raw Juice Therapy, Thorsons Editorial Board, Thorsons, 1989.

Keane, Maureen B., *Juicing for Good Health*, Pocket Books, 1992.

Kenton, Leslie and Susannah, *Raw Energy*, Arrow, 1986.

Kordich, Jay, *The Juiceman's Power of Juicing*, Morrow, 1992.

Nutrition

Calorie Counter, Collins Gem, HarperCollins, 1991.

Chaitow, Leon, *The Stress Protection Plan*, Thorsons, 1992

———, *Clear Body, Clear Mind*, Thorsons, 1990.

Davies, Dr Stephen and Dr Alan Stewart, *Nutritional Medicine*, Pan, 1987.

Kunz-Bircher, Ruth, *The Bircher-Benner Health Guide*, Allen and Unwin, 1981.

Mindell, Earl, *The Vitamin Bible*, Arlington, 1979.

Newhouse, Sonia, *Complete Natural Food Facts*, Thorsons, 1991.

Pauling, Linus, *How To Live Longer and Feel Better*, W.H. Freeman and Company, 1986.

Vogel, Dr. H.C.A., *The Nature Doctor*, Mainstream, 1990.

Therapies *(with reference to Chapter 7)*

Aromatherapy: Shirley Price, *Practical Aromatherapy*, Thorsons, 1987

Beauty treatments: Anita Guyton, *The Natural Beauty Book*, Thorsons, 1991.

Massage: Clare Maxwell-Hudson, *The Complete Book of Massage*, Dorling Kindersley, 1989

Relaxation: Simon Brown and Dan Fletcher, *Vital Touch*, Community Health Foundation, 1991.

index

aches and pains 76-8
acid-alkaline balance 7, 104
acne 58-9
additives 106
alertness 89-90
alfalfa 9, 31
allergic rhinitis 64-5
Al's super zinger 134
amino acids 3, 104
anaemia 81-2
antioxidants 5
aphrodisiacs 100-1
apples 15, 114, 115
   apple whizz 151
apricots 16
   apricot, nut and plum teabread 190
   apricot smoothie 132
aromatherapy massage 120
arthritis 76-7
asthma 64-5
avocados 16-17, 49
   avocado smoothie 152

bad breath 69
bananas 17, 49
   banana bounty 137
   banana daiquiri 162
   banana passion 133
   banana and pear shake 131
bartender's breakfast 159-60
beansprouts 9, 32, 127-9
beetnik 146
beetroot 32, 114, 115, 147
   beetroot slammer 141
belle des poires 159
berries
   berry punch 165

berry smoothie 130
berry yoghurt 187
beta-carotene 4, 51
bioflavinoids 3
blackberries 17-18
   blackberry hollow 150
blackcurrants 18
blemishes 105
blended fruit 127
blondie 161
blood pressure 50
blood sugar 8
blueberries 18-19
   blueberry blast 138
body scrunching 121
body-brushing 104, 119
Boston blue punch 164
breakfast 111, 116, 118, 139-43
breathing 60
bright eyes 149
broccoli 33
bronchitis 62-3
brown rice salad 181
Brussels sprouts 33
burns 66
buying produce 13-14

cabbage 34-5
cakes 189-90
calcium 85
calmness 90-1
candidiasis 8, 50, 104, 107
Caribbean milk shake 135
carrots 35, 114
   carrot and banana cake 189
   carrot and coriander 144
   carrot and orange soup 167

carrot smoothie 132

carrot zinger 141

catarrh 105

cauliflowers 36

celeriac 36

celery 37

centrifugal juicers 10

cherries 19

children 13, 49, 107

   recipes 147-52

chilli bean pot 176

chlorophyll 6, 60, 127

Christmas cranberry 146

citrus fruits 9, 125

   squeezers 11

cleaning juicers 12

cleansing 2, 6-7, 50, 99-100, 103, 107, 110, 116

cocktails 129, 153-63

coconut 127

colds 60, 61-2

constipation 71-2

cool carrot 146

coughs 62-3

cramp 67

cranberries 19-20

   cranberry twist 147

crispy red cabbage and apple salad 180

cucumbers 37

   cucumber and avocado lassi 136-7

   cucumber combo 144

curly kale 151

customizing juices 125-9

cystitis 82-3

dandruff 53-4

degenerative disease 79-80

delicious fig 139

detox programmes 6-7, 56, 103-23

diabetes 50, 107

diarrhoea 72-3

digestion 6, 49, 68-75, 104-5, 110, 112, 116

dilution 7, 13, 49, 129, 147

elderly, see old age

energy 95

Epsom salt baths 119-20

equipment 11, 205

exercise 106

exotic fruit punch 165

eyes 51-2

facial steams 121

fatigue 93-4

fennel 38

fibre 3, 6, 71

fire eater 157

flatulence 8, 50

flu 63-4

food processors 9

free radicals 5

fructose 8

fruit 105, 107, 116

   blended 127

   buying 13-14

   preparation 15-31

garlic 38

gentle grapefruit 145

golden carrot 140

gooseberries 20

grapefruit 21, 114

   grapefruit sun splash 151

grapes 20-1

   grape ripple 140

   grapeberry 155

green wonder 132

greengages 21-2

greensleeves 158

guavas 22

guidelines 50

hair 52-4, 122

hangovers 96-7
happy apple 152
hay fever 64-5
headaches 77-8, 105
herbs 49, 126
herby carrot burgers 171
honey 49, 126
honey bee 155
hydraulic juice presses 10

ice-cream 126
indigestion 70-1
insomnia 92
Irritable Bowel Syndrome 73-4

Joe cool 157-8

kale 39
kiwis 22-3
   king kiwi 140
   kiwi cooler 143
kudos special 158-9

leeks 39
lemons 23
   lemon chicken stir-fry 178
lettuce 40
limes 23-4
liquidizers 9
lunch 111, 116, 118
lymphatic system 104
magnesium 68, 85
main courses 169-79
mangetout 40
mangos 24
   mango carrot 152
   mango chicken 169
   mango milkshake 133
   mango and peach lassi 136
   mango tango smoothie 150
manicures 121-2

massage 104, 120
masticating juicers 10
meditation 106, 121
melons 24-5
   melon refresher 145
menopause 85-6
migraines 77-8
milk 126
minerals 2, 3, 3-5, 15, 49, 51, 97-8, 104, 106,
   191, 196-200
Mississippi mule 156
mixed berry crumble 184
mixed fruit and veg salad 182
multi-vitamin/mineral boost 98-9

nails 54-5
nausea 74-5
nectarines 25
nerves 96
nose-cone pressure juicers 10
nutty stuffed peppers 170

old age 101-2, 107
One Day Juice Plan 104-8, 110-12
One Week Vitality Plan 104-8, 113-23, 205
onions 41
oranges 25-6
   orange, banana and raspberry smoothie 137
   orange blossom 161
   orange punch 164
   orange and raspberry sherbet 188
organic produce 13-14
osteoporosis 85

pampering 104, 110, 113, 119-23
papayas 26
   papaya smoothie 130-1
parsley 9, 41, 147
parsnip 42
passion fruits 26-7
passion juice 131

pasta with bacon and celery 177
Paul's mai tai 160
peaches 27
    peach and banana brûlée 186
    peach daiquiri 162
    peaches 'n' cream 153-4
    peachy sweet 135, 136
peak papaya 144
pears 27-8
    pear drop 143
peppers 42
    pepper up 142
phosphorus 4
pina colada 155
pineapples 28
    pineapple and banana smoothie 150
    pineapple and pear perfection 130
in the pink 138
pink mango 131
planter's punch 162–3
plums 28-9
pollution 103-4
potassium 4, 49, 51
potatoes 43
prawn and mango filo parcels 173
pregnancy 84-5
Premenstrual Syndrome (PMS) 83-4
professional help 107, 202-4
puddings 183-8
pulp 10, 12, 126, 166-90
punches 163-5

quantity guide 108-9
quick cleanse 99-100

radishes 43
raspberries 29
    raspberry sparkle 149
recipes
    breakfast 139-43
    cakes 189-90

    children 147-52
    cocktails 153-63
    lunch 144-5
    main course 169-79
    One Week Vitality Plan 114-15
    puddings 183-8
    pulp 166-90
    punches 163-5
    salads 180-2
    smoothies 130-9
    starters 167-8
    supper 145-7
    vitamin/mineral boost 98-9
red cabbage 34
red wine spaghetti 174
redhead 159
relaxation techniques 106
respiration 60
rheumatism 76-7
Ritz fizz 163
rules 7-8

St Clement's 142
salads 180-2
salt rubs 104, 119
saunas 104, 120
scalds 66
Sergeant pepper 145
sex life 100-1
shades of summer 134
shopping 13-14, 110, 113
simply strawberry 144
sitting pretty 154
skin 55-9
smoothie recipes 130-9
snacks 117
snow peas 40
sodium 67
sore throats 61-2
soya shake 134
specialist suppliers 10, 205

spices 49, 126
  spicy spinach pâté 168
  spicy vegetable couscous 172
spinach 44, 114, 147
sprouts, see beansprouts
starters 167-8
stomach ulcers 94-5
strawberries 29-30
  strawberry daiquiri 157
  strawberry fields 160
  strawberry ice 133
stress 90-1
super A 138
super carrot 143, 152
supper 111, 116, 118, 145-7
sweet dreams 154
sweet pear 149
sweet potatoes 44-5
sweet and sour pork 175
sweetness and light 158

tangerines 30
  tangerine tickler 150
tangy lemon and lime mousse 183
teenagers 147, 148
Thai spice 141-2
Thai-style fish casserole 179
thrush 8
tips 12-13
tomatoes 45
  tomato bliss 143
  tomato toner 146
  tomato topper 151
Turkish baths 104, 120
turnips 45-6

typhoon 154-5

ulcers 94-5

vegetables 105, 107, 116
  buying 13-14
  preparation 31-47
Virgin Mary 156
vitamins 2, 3, 3-5, 12, 15, 49, 51, 98-9, 104, 106, 191-6
vomiting 74-5

Walker, N. 3
warrior punch 163
water 106, 129
water retention 86
watercress 46-7, 147
  watercress whizz 142
watermelons 30-1
  watermelon wonder 149
weight-loss 75-6, 107
wheatgerm 49, 127
wheatgrass 9
white cabbage 35
wholewheat crêpes with peach sauce 185
winter cabbage 34
withdrawal symptoms 105
women 80-7
wounds 87-8
wrinkle-busters 57-8

yoga 106
yoghurt 49, 126, 187

zinc 51